S0-AEO-518

Health and Medical Care in the U.S.:

A CRITICAL ANALYSIS

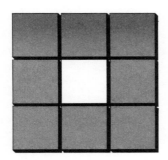

Theodore Lownik Library
Illinois Benedictine College
Lisle, Illinois 60532

Health and Medical Care in the U.S.:

A CRITICAL ANALYSIS

Edited by Vicente Navarro

**POLICY,
POLITICS,
HEALTH AND
MEDICINE**

Series

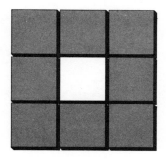

Baywood Publishing Company, Inc.

Farmingdale, N.Y.   11735

362.1
P766
v. 1

Copyright © 1973, 1974, 1975 in the International Journal of Health Services by Baywood Publishing Company, Inc., Farmingdale, New York. All rights reserved. Printed in the United States of America.

Library of Congress Catalog Card Number: 77-70380

ISBN Number: 0-89503-000-4

© Copyright 1977, Baywood Publishing Company, Inc.

Health and Medical Care in the U.S.:
A CRITICAL ANALYSIS

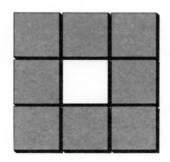

PREFACE

The essays in this collection aim at challenging the prevalent interpretations and understandings of health, medicine and medical care in our Western capitalist societies in general and in North America in particular, as well as at providing alternative explanations for those realities. And although a diversity of positions are represented in the collection, each article shares a commonality of purpose: the presentation of a critique of those well-established ideologies that are rooted in orthodoxy and terra firma. Originally published in the *International Journal of Health Services*—a quarterly committed to a plurality of opinion within its pages—the essays have been selected because they present a radical critique of the medical care sector that, in our Weberian-monopolized sociological world, demands exposure and deserves debate.

The first of the volume's four parts, Part I, presents three articles which challenge the utilitarian, positivist and functionalist visions of health (Kelman's) and medicine (Frankenberg's), as well as their political interpretations and uses (Navarro's). Kelman's essay, which opens the series, has stirred considerable controversy since its publication in the *International Journal of Health Services*. Challenging the prevalent ahistorical interpretations of health, Kelman counterposes an historical materialist approach and details the operational implications of such an approach for present-day U.S. society. Frankenberg criticizes several paradigms that are (and historically have been) influential in medical sociology circles, using Marx (rather than Weber) as his point of departure. In the last article in this part, I make a critique of the ideological construct that is most frequently used to explain the nature of our Western developed societies, i.e., industrialism. Considering Ivan Illich as one of its main theorists, I review his assumptions and challenge his political conclusions, positing that it is capitalism, not industrialism, that determines the nature of our societies and subsequently of our systems of medicine.

Part II includes three articles which aim at imparting a specific understanding of medical care in the U.S. within the political and economic parameters of late capitalism. In his widely-cited contribution, Bodenheimer analyzes the ways in which the system of funding of health care in the U.S. reflects the overall pattern of dominance of our political institutions by the wealthy and the powerful—a dominance that determines highly skewed and inequitable fiscal policies and systems of funding from which the medical care sector is not insulated. This approach to the political and economic forces in our society is further developed and detailed in the other two articles in this part. Bodenheimer, Cummings and Harding analyze the health insurance industry and the consequences for the medical sector of its dominant position. My article examines the health sector of the U.S., viewing it as the dialectical result of the overall class relations in our society.

Part III includes Fee's article which analyzes the three main forces presently existing within the U.S. feminist movement and provides a point of entry for discussion of strategies for change towards the resolution of the longest march of all.

In all these articles, and in their quest for the redefinition of health and medicine, emphasis is placed on the need for profound change in the economic, political and social structures of our society and the relations they determine. And in that analysis and in that quest, the role of the state—the subject of Renaud's article (Part IV)—is a key one. In his article, Renaud challenges the belief held by the pluralists and power elite analysts that the state is neutral and is thus the proper *champ de bataille* for change. He postulates instead that the state intervention is integrally linked to the pattern of capital accumulation and class relations which determine the nature of the constraints imposed in that intervention.

The essays in this volume, then, within their individual diversity, combine to direct a challenge to the ideologies and beliefs that predominate in the medical care sector. It is their intention to question the stifling patterns of analytical orthodoxy which simply replicate the class, race and sex relations in our society. And the commonality of their intention is that of providing new interpretations of health, medicine and medical care as the first step towards changing them.

Vicente Navarro
Johns Hopkins University

TABLE OF CONTENTS

PART 1

The Definition of
Health and Medicine.

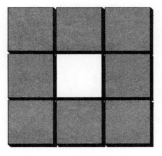

CHAPTER 1

The Social Nature of the Definition of Health

Sander Kelman

Perhaps the most perplexing and ambiguous issue in the study of health since its inception centuries or millenia ago, is its definition. Currently, most curricula in the study of public health devote a certain, nominal, amount of time to the issue, reviewing definitions offered by earlier writers, but the conclusion is always that the definitions have virtually no operational or empirical significance, and, more importantly, that the definition question is not problematic to the empirical analysis of epidemiology, health care institutions, and health care policy. In general the issue is obviated by assuming, either implicitly or explicitly, that "health" is the absence of illness.

In this chapter it is argued that through adoption of the appropriate theoretical approach and the derivation of suitable analytical categories, the definition problem can be seen as operational, nontrivial, and highly problematic to the determination of health care policy. More concretely, the chapter attempts to isolate the social basis of the definition of health (hereafter, "health," to distinguish from the word health, without quotation marks, which will signify *health status*). Put another way, the principal focus here is on the social origins of the adoption of particular norms, notions, or dimensions of organismic well-being, and not primarily on the social causes of illness itself.

Schematically, the first part of the chapter (Theoretical Derivation) develops the theoretical approach to the problem. It begins with Kuhn's approach to the understanding of scientific development, an approach that views scientific progress as arising primarily out of scholarly debate within the particular scientific profession in question. This approach is illustrated with the development of thinking in the field of the psychology of intelligence, and then applied to the definition problem in health, generating a proposed new set of categories for resolving the definition problem.

Analytically, however, this is not sufficient, since the principal problem in the sociology of knowledge is the understanding of the social and historical context in which certain ideas, attitudes, and norms of behavior arise or do not arise, not simply the ex post chronicling of the intellectual activities of the academic parties to the dispute. The latter section of part one, therefore, elaborates a historical materialist theoretical framework to derive the same conclusion generated out of Kuhn's approach. Part one concludes with a critical review of existing definitions of health and a discussion of the possibilities of an analytically valid normative conception of health.

The second part (Application of the Theory) applies the new definition by reinterpreting parts of the history of public health and medicine, and concludes with a discussion of how this definition is highly problematic to the major structural reforms currently under way in the American health care system.

THEORETICAL DERIVATION

Thomas Kuhn in his now-celebrated book, *The Structure of Scientific Revolutions* (1), argues that the principal characteristic of any field of scientific inquiry during any particular epoch in its development is the fundamental *paradigm* (postulate) that organizes the practice of "normal science" during that epoch. Hence, astronomy, some 500 years ago, passed from the paradigm of geocentrism to that of heliocentrism and beyond.

Yet, if one were to inquire about the fundamental paradigm currently in practice in the study of health, silence would likely follow. At the very most, social scientists, whose primary orientation is disciplinary (e.g. economics or sociology), rather than substantive (e.g. health), would respond with paradigms from their respective disciplines: moral hazard, (sick) role, pluralism, and so forth. To move closer still, pathology and medicine do have their own paradigms, but like those imposed from social science, beg the substantive issues of "health" itself.

If there is anything to the framework elaborated by Kuhn, however, there is, in past and contemporary research and thinking on "health," an identifiable paradigm transcending medicine and social science, but implicit within their applications in the study of "health."

The purpose and direction of this section, then, is to identify the recent paradigm development in "health," propose a new paradigm, and discover the historical genesis of its real-world counterpart.

To first gain some intellectual distance on the subject, however, a brief look at the development of paradigm structures in the psychology of intelligence is presented. In the discussion of paradigm development of both "intelligence"[1] and "health," a three-stage sequence is uncovered: universal-mechanistic, asocial developmental, and social developmental.

The classical paradigm in the study of intelligence (Binet) was that of a universal, genetically fixed endowment of cognitive capacity—specifically, the innate ability to solve extrinsically defined problems. That is, "intelligence" (according to this paradigm) was (and is) assumed to be *qualitatively* invariant across culture and secularly

---

[1] As in the case of "health," "intelligence" will be taken to mean the particular form(s) of cognitive competence adopted in particular societies or assumed as paradigmatic in psychological study. Intelligence (without quotation marks) will denote the empirical achievement of that competence.

invariant through societies over time; moreover, in a particular individual, cognitive *capacity* was assumed to be largely fixed genetically, and the degree of its achievement was determined by the individual's social and cultural context. Intelligence testing, at its best, was aimed at measuring the endowment of such "intelligence," whereas learning theory, and, in its more applied form, schooling, are assumed to be directed at the attempt to achieve the maximum use of the differentially distributed, but qualitatively universal, cognitive capacity.

Beginning with Piaget, however, the validity of the notion of "intelligence" as an analytic entity having a real empirical correspondent is no longer universally accepted. Instead, according to Piaget and his followers, "intelligence" is merely a continuous interaction between perception and cognition, each in its turn altering the other (2).

Whereas Piaget's contribution lies in his apparently correct recognition that "intelligence" is not an endowed entity, the weakness of his viewpoint, and that of his followers, lies in their view of "intelligence" as a universal process. That is, his lifetime of research has been devoted to verifying that in all societies the same stages of cognitive development are experienced. In sum, whereas the scholars of the Binet school perceive "intelligence" as a universal entity, Piaget and his followers see it as a universal process, similar in all societies, culminating, as one psychologist has put it, in the form of Swiss scientist (3).

Over much the same period as the development of Piaget's work, a third group of psychologists has, in effect, attempted to supplant his paradigm and pursue empirical research on the premise that "the fundamental categories of psychological processes in man are of an historical character and that psychology must be understood as an historical science . . ." (4).

> [O]ver the past 70 years there have been sporadic but recurrent assertions of the notion that people raised in different cultures are different intellectually, have different cognitive competences. These assertions appear to go beyond the usually accepted notion of *quantitative* differences on a single, universal cognitive dimension, to the notion that there are *qualitatively* differing cognitive competences appropriate to the requirements of a particular culture. Whether all peoples have access to all dimensions (but produce a different *pattern* of scores on them), or some peoples have access to some *unique* dimensions, is immaterial; what matters is the assertion of more than a single universal dimension called (in the West) "intelligence" (5, p. 83; emphasis in original).

Continuing on this tack, then, the scientific effort is directed to the identification of the *"qualitatively* differing cognitive competences" and, most important, to the understanding of the mechanism by which different societal forms generate and promote different "cognitive competences." Since the present task is not the elaboration of the development of intelligence psychology, but rather the demonstration that what is to be argued in the case of "health" has its analytical counterparts elsewhere in social science, the discussion of "intelligence" is here ended.

Paradigm Development in Health

In a similar fashion, but in more detail, the development of thinking in the field of health can be understood. Although discussions of the nature of "health" go back at least to the work of Galen, this discussion begins with the transition from religious to scientific orientations in the conception of "health" and disease.

The first apparent scientific paradigm for health originated with the development of the machine model of the human body (since the mind or soul was relegated to a separate compartment). With this conception, "health" came to be seen as the perfect working order of the human organism, likening the human organism to an automaton (a self-propelling machine) (6). Moreover, the methodologies of pathology and diagnostics that developed from this view (and continue to dominate in the practice of medicine, today) consider illness to be both natural (biological) and occurring on an individual basis. Treatment, therefore, is pursued on an individual bio-chemo-surgical basis, relegating the recognition and implications of social causes of illness to secondary importance, though even this secondary recognition must be viewed as "ad hoc modification" (1, p. 78) in the face of the next paradigm to be discussed.

Although the recognition of the social basis of many diseases and ill health goes far back in medical history, the greatest boost probably came with the publication of the Chadwick Report in England and the Shattuck Report in the United States in the mid-19th century. Since that time there has been a great deal of writing on social epidemiology and the environmentalist approach to health, and this represents the second major paradigm in the discussion of health, for it is clearly in conflict with the biological and individual orientation of the classical school, still very much the predominant methodology. Yet the purpose of this paper is to show that even if their differences could be resolved, the substance of "health" is still not defined.

The parallel between the social epidemiologists and the Piaget school is quite striking. Both go beyond bio-individualism in recognizing that both "health" and "intelligence" arise out of developmental processes in which the individual interacts with the social environment. Both, however, generally assume the respective process and "health" and "intelligence" themselves to be universal—independent of the form of society in which they are investigated. Whereas Piaget normatively conceives of intelligence as the highest stage of a universal cognitive competence, the social epidemiologists, accordingly, conceive of health as a lack of breakdown in a universal notion of human organismic integrity. As discussed above, this assumption is being seriously challenged in the psychology of intelligence; the purpose of the remainder of this paper is to mount the same challenge in the field of "health."

Paradigm and Anomaly in "Health"

The central feature of discussions about the transition from one paradigm to another (Kuhn's "Scientific Revolution") is the existence of *anomaly:* evidence that tends to invalidate the prevailing paradigm in use in the current practice of the science. Consider evidence anomalous to the mechanistic, individual paradigm that originated with Descartes and Harvey. Given the machine model and analytic compartmentalization and disposal of emotional processes that are a continuing theme in medical science today, there is no accounting for the wealth of anomalous evidence on placebo effects, voodoo-induced death, and other psychosomatic illnesses. Their methodology is simply too limited to incorporate the circumscription of the physical aspects of existence by the social dimensions of consciousness (7). At most these psychosomatic processes are relegated to the category of emotional stressors that disturb the homeostatic equilibrium of the body (8, pp. 4-5). This tends to externalize emotional processes from the biochemistry of the body, thereby reducing them to a conception of etiology consistent with the germ theory of disease. It also transforms emotional and social processes into temporary perturbations of a basic biological state, rather than constant strong determinants of it. Once again, this must be seen as the ad hoc modification of theory (1, p. 78).

To generalize, the bio-individual school encounters major difficulty whenever it seeks to impose a generalized germ theory on a pathology the etiology of which is a complex dialectic between the organism and socially induced stresses. The current thrust of cancer research toward the end of isolating a cancer virus, with a view to subsequently developing the appropriate antibody, is probably such a case of misplaced methodology. Similarly, the use of psychosurgery to curb violent behavior, on the assumption that that behavior results from a focal organic brain dysfunction, rather than from the social conditions of the violent, reproduces this positivist methodology.

Whereas the advances of the social epidemiology school over the science of its predecessor lie in the area of etiology, it still suffers from the implicit assumption that "health" itself is biologically, not socially, determined, that the substantive meaning of "health" is not a variant. Although psychologists have begun to recognize the existence of "qualitatively differing cognitive competences," it does not appear that health scholarship has begun to recognize "qualitatively differing organismic integrities."

This anomaly becomes apparent when the extent to which symptom-masking passes for disease treatment is recognized. The etiology of heart disease and stroke is recognized, even in the leading medical journals, to be bound up in the social organization and dynamics in which its victims live (9), yet this view does not receive coherent formulation and application to cure. Despite the available evidence, the bio-individual school formulates the causes as genetic, while the social epidemiological school extends the assignment of etiology only a few steps further to diet, smoking, obesity, or "life style," that is to things that mediate the ultimate social causes. Both schools agree on treatment as well: administration of screening, chemotherapy, and heart operations to mitigate the effects of hypertension, the proximate cause.

Similarly, cancers are today recognized to result, in 60-90 per cent of the cases, from artificially created, environmental carcinogens (10), yet the prescribed treatment is ex post radiation, chemotherapy, and surgical removal rather than environmental prevention. Although, "normal" mental illness (depression, chronic anxiety, etc.) is similarly recognized to result from adverse social organization (11), again, the prescribed treatment is some combination of drugs, psychotherapy, transcendental meditation, and other forms of instrumental, victim-blaming "cures."

Such scientific emphasis on attempted cure, rather than prevention, might be scientifically justifiable in terms of the limited state of our understanding of the etiology of these diseases *were there also a major and visible discussion and research effort directed toward the social reorganization necessary to prevent these leading causes of illness and death.* In its absence, however, the inevitable conclusion must be that there are at least two fundamental and conflicting notions or dimensions of "health": *experiential* and *functional.* The former may be defined as freedom from illness, the capacity for human development and self-discovery, and the transcendence of alienating social circumstances. Given the above treatment modes, it falls in the face of the latter: the "state of optimum *capacity* of an individual for the effective performance of the roles and tasks for which he has been socialized" (12, p. 117). The two are quite different concretely, in terms of the respective "health" policies that they imply, and in what remains the relationship between the mode of social organization and the particular "health" policy will be discussed. Moreover, they are substantially in conflict given that health policies established upon the experiential definition of "health" would suggest the elimination of those social conditions that give rise to illness, whereas policies established upon the functional definition may merely suggest either the intervention between the social stressors and their associated pathogenesis (as through drugs) or the ex post treatment of those illnesses (as through surgery). Stated another way, experiential health refers to *intrinsically* defined organismic integrity, whereas functional health refers to *extrinsically* defined organismic integrity.

To return to the point of departure, it will be argued that a new paradigm in the science of health must be adopted: one that recognizes that health behavior, in any society, is socially determined even to the extent that "health" itself is primarily socially, rather than strictly biologically, determined; it is largely a socially determined category predicated upon the particular characteristics and dynamics of the society under investigation. In sum, experiential and functional health represent two qualitatively differing notions or norms of organismic integrity which are either promoted or stunted in different forms of society.

The Materialist Approach to the Study of Health

The development of this third paradigm (that "health" itself is socially defined) can begin with the axiom that human beings are the basis of both the forces of production (physical ingredients of production, such as labor, resources, and equipment) and the relations of production (division of labor, legal, property, and social institutions and practices) in any society, and that therefore "appropriate human organismic condition" (i.e. "health") can only be understood in the concrete context of the particular mode of organization of production and the dialectical relationship between the productive forces and relations (13). Hence, in a society in which the system of production tends to dominate the pattern and dynamics of social organization, rather than vice versa, it can be expected that experiential health would tend to wane in the face of the more "appropriate" functional health.

Specifically, in the United States where production is privately owned and directed, and the apparatus of the state is often dominated by the interests of private capital, the sordid history of occupational illness and death (14, 15) emerges in labor surplus situations as a mechanism of imposing certain costs of production onto the work force, rather than onto shareholders or customers. In the same general context, when labor is in relatively short supply or the costs of labor replacement are high, the "unhealthiness" of the work environment is not so severe. In either case, "health" is subordinated to production rather than an end in itself, and it is under these circumstances that the category of functional "health" has concrete significance.

In the discussion which follows, "health" is analyzed in the context of a specific form of society—capitalist society—and is seen to depend heavily on the theory of alienation.

Capitalist Society. The immediate distinguishing features of capitalist societies, in contrast with feudal or socialist, are that production takes place within markets and is encouraged by the ability of private producers to sell their products or services for more than their costs of production (profit). For the purpose of the discussion which follows, however, a more fundamental understanding of capitalist social dynamics is necessary.

First, individual producers, whether small firms or giant corporations, generally compete with others in the same line of business. Hence, from the point of view of the individual producer, survival is an immediate and overwhelming consideration. Survival, and the continued capacity to generate profits, thereby sets in motion two prominent derivative concerns: the expansion of markets and the reduction of costs. This is so because every individual producer is aware that every other individual producer in the same market is concerned about survival and is consequently driven toward market expansion and cost reduction so as to avoid being beaten by the competition. If they do not engage in these practices, there is always the fear that others will, and they will lose.

With most firms operating in this type of environment, then, economic growth is a necessary correlate of such a society. This is so because both the expansion of individual markets and the reduction of costs generally require the continual expansion of productive facilities, as well as the development and emplacement of new cost-cutting technologies.

This expansion, or, in the aggregate, the accumulation of capital, takes place through the generation and diversion of social savings (corporate retained earnings and personal savings) to the financing of productive expansion. Given that capitalist commerce is today internationalized, this thrust toward accumulation cannot easily be constrained, since it would then place the entire national economy in jeopardy for reasons similar to those requiring individual producers in a market to expand.

Hence, given the private ownership and control of the basic institutions of production, this process of accumulation operates largely outside of whatever democratic political institutions exist and can never be considered the subject of social choice. Moreover, as a consequence, the division of labor, the nature of work, the level of technology, the pace of automation, the degree of environmental abuse, the available forms of transportation, the thrust of schooling and education, urbanization, foreign policy, etc., etc., all tend to be derivative of the underlying thrust toward and patterns of private accumulation, rather than independent, democratic, social choices.

To be sure, there is a theory dominant in neoclassical economics which argues that production through profit incentives and markets is validated and thereby justified by consumer demand.

Based in utilitarian theory, however, this pretense of normative consumer demand is merely metaphysical since it does not consider the social and historical fashion in which consumer demand is generated, and instead relegates the discussion to multi-dimensional, metaphysical utility functions. And in those (many) cases where demand is itself directly created by the activities of those who stand ready to fulfil it (the suppliers, i.e. auto industry, medical care (16)), this neoclassical theory becomes even worse than metaphysical, namely ideological. The preceding can be summarized in the following definition:

> *Capitalism* is a social system in which social institutions and their develop-
> ment and the social identity and role of the individual are subordinated to
> the largely autonomous process of capital accumulation, generally, but not
> always, in the context of the private ownership of that capital.[2]

[2]It is today increasingly agreed that the Soviet Union and its East European satellites, despite the absence of the private ownership of the means of production, are more accurately depicted as state capitalist rather than socialist countries, as defined below. There, as in the West, the social development since the 1920s has tended to be subordinated to industrialization and the accumulation of capital. To be sure, the dynamics that set this in motion are quite different from those in the West (arising instead from the managerial class, which controls both the production system and the state) and take their cues for the direction of development from the (capitalist) West.

Some examples will help to amplify this definition. First, there is Fromm's secular analysis of human personality under capitalism (11, pp. 76-184). In it Fromm demonstrates how the dominant personality modes are conditioned by the structural modes of production. Specifically, where self-employment is the dominant pattern in a mass society (up to the early part of the present century) rugged individualism appears to have been the dominant socially approved personality mode. As the structure of production and accumulation became ever more concentrated and self-employment ceased to be the dominant pattern, however, the personality mode of the organization man with all of its attributes of deference and repression (17) came to supplant that of the rugged individualist. It is probably correct that such a transition was never the express object of any public or private policy. However, it was informally disciplined by the organizational dismissal of people who "can't get along with others." What this illustration does demonstrate is that the accumulation and concentration of capital proceed on their own (largely autonomous) logic, and personality and social relations are forced to adjust.

A second, though not wholly separate, example is that of the origins of public schooling. Very briefly, with the rise of the factory system of production and the wage system of payment, came a new system of institutions for the socialization of the young.

> An ideal preparation for the factory work was found in the social relations of the school: specifically, in its emphasis on discipline, punctuality, acceptance of authority outside the family, and individual accountability for one's work. The social relations of the school would replicate the social relations of the work place, and thus help young people adapt to the social division of labor. Schools would further lead people to accept the authority of the state and its agents—the teachers—at a young age, in part by fostering the illusion of the benevolence of the government in its relations with citizens. Moreover, because schooling would ostensibly be open to all, one's position in the division of labor could be portrayed as the result not of birth, but of one's own efforts and talents ... (18, p. 221).

Said a Lowell textile manufacturer, writing to Horace Mann, Secretary of the Massachusetts Board of Education, in 1841:

> I have never considered mere knowledge ... as the only advantage derived from a good ... education .... [Workers with more education] are more orderly and respectful in their deportment, and more ready to comply with the wholesome and necessary regulations of an establishment .... In times of agitation I have always looked to the most intelligent, best educated and the most moral for support. The ignorant and uneducated I have generally found the most turbulent and troublesome, acting under the impulse of excited passion and jealousy (19, p. 38).

In this case the adjustment process is very much the express policy of the state (18-22).

A third example concerns more recent "policies" regarding this same dialectic. A great deal has been written over the past two decades tracing the social etiology of much of the neurosis, psychosis, and alienation to the very social cement of Western industrialized nations: competition (23, 24). In particular, the construction of social relations on an adversary, rather than cooperative, basis (another important function of public education) generates a wet-finger-to-the-wind sense of identity which often comes into conflict with more authentic internal needs. In mild cases this leads to various forms of neurosis and in extreme cases to schizophrenia. Consequently, what we have witnessed over the past two decades is the proliferation of various modes of chemical and psychomanipulative maintenance, which deal, literally, with symptoms, rather than causes. One need only peruse the pages of any American medical or public health journal to quickly recognize the "solution" to mood and depression problems offered by the Pharmaceutical Manufacturers Association. Or one can choose among a variety of brands of victim-blaming psychological and psychiatric counseling techniques which do not recognize and deal with the manner in which personality contradictions are tied up in the social relations of production over which the victim has little control. Or in desperation one can opt for the approach of the new wave of lobotomists currently being encouraged and/or enticed by substantial grants from the National Institute of Mental Health[3] and the Law Enforcement Assistance Administration of the Department of Justice (25). Some of these "solutions" are express policies of social control; others, indeed most, are, once again, merely survival-induced adjustment processes. What is critical, however, is that these are the range of choices available to people, given the autonomous process of capital accumulation and the social context in which it proceeds.

To that brief discussion of the social and economic dynamics of capitalist society is appended a definition of socialist society, intended strictly for the purposes of analytical clarity, not social interpretation:

> *Socialism* is a social system in which the production system (capital accumulation) is subordinated to, though not independent of, the democratically determined process and direction of social development.[4]

A further category, central to this discussion, is that of objectification:

> *Objectification* is the process of psychological adjustment to and institutionalized control over individuals by capitalist (as defined above) development.

Putting the definitions of capitalism and objectification together, then, objectification is the system of controls over individuals and their consciousness by institutions not ultimately, even collectively, controllable by them. Crudely put, *objectification* is the process by which and the context in which people become the objects of their social system.

A final definition is that of alienation:

> *Alienation* is the existential, not psychological, situation in which individuals do not exert ultimate control, either individually or collectively, over their social world.

Several points of clarification need to be made here. First, it is *not* required by this definition of alienation that people be aware of it. It is an "objective" situation, not a state of awareness. It does, however, have serious psychological implications and consequences (24, 26, 27).

Consistent variations of this theme are those of Fromm: the experience of oneself as the object, rather than the subject, of one's existence (11, p. 111); and Marx: the situation in which people make choices, but not on their own terms (rather "under circumstances directly encountered, given, and transmitted from the past") (28, p. 15).

---

[3] At this writing, temporarily discontinued.

[4] No doubt, this definition will anger both Marxists and non-Marxists. For the latter, this definition inaccurately depicts existing "socialist" societies; for the former, it confuses socialism with communism. Both objections are correct. The purpose of this discussion of capitalism, socialism, and alienation is merely to provide an analytical framework within which to discuss the definition of health, not primarily to evaluate existing societies.

It should be clear that objectification and alienation are largely the same thing seen from opposite ends of the telescope: the former from the point of view of the "system," its architects and managers themselves, perhaps, alienated, and the latter from the point of view of the objectified population.

"Health" in Capitalist Society. It is now possible to insert the discussion of "health" into the framework of alienation. At any point in time functional "health" is that organismic condition of the population most consistent with, or least disruptive of, the process of capital accumulation. At the individual level this means the capacity to effectively do productive (contributing to accumulation) work. In the aggregate a population is said to be functionally healthy if the expenditures necessary to bring that condition about are not so high as to interfere with the expansion of capital. More precisely, a population is said to be optimally functionally healthy if the last increment of resources directed toward health contributes as much to overall productivity and accumulation as it would if diverted toward direct capital investment (accumulation). To be sure, such a policy cannot always be operationalized completely, particularly when cultural patterns interfere. For example, this policy would suggest the termination of health care resources to the nonproductive: the aged, the chronically unemployed, and the catastrophically ill. To date, in the West, such policies are not, in the strict sense, politically viable, although such a direction is suggested by continuing statements emanating from the executive branch of the U.S. government to the effect that resources currently being allocated to social and governmental services must be redirected toward private investment if the economy is to get back on its feet.

Moreover, to the extent that the substantial social elimination of competition (and, therefore, anxiety, stress, and insecurity) and the elimination of environmental and occupational carcinogens and other pathogens, would severely interfere with the context in which accumulation takes place, that elimination would have to be viewed as lying outside the realm of an "appropriate" functional health policy. In any case, functional "health" suggests a very explicit, empirical, and operational thrust to health care policy in a capitalist society (as defined above). Further, the alienating consequences of such a policy are quite evident.

Experiential health, on the other hand, grows more out of the relations of production than it does from the forces of production, which largely elicit the functional definition of health, but experiential health must still be conceptualized within the framework of alienation. Experiential health is simply people's own conception of what it is to be "healthy," and this conception may vary widely with respect to objective accuracy. To the extent that people's conception is inaccurate, relative to the existing state of (accurate) health knowledge, and to the extent that people (often have no choice but to) act contrary to their own self-interested health knowledge (stress, environmental carcinogens, occupational disease), and to the extent that their experience and capacity for fulfillment and self-development are truncated by their unhealthy means of coping with alienating circumstances (alcohol and drug addiction), then for that society, class, or individual, experiential health is an empirical subject in the study of alienation. A final assumption, then, is that the less alienating a society is, the more control individuals exert over their social circumstances, both individually and collectively, the less alienating are their notions and practices of experiential "health" likely to be.

Consequently, in a capitalist society with continual conflicts between the accumulation process and the process of social development, there are two inherent social contradictions in the definition of health: that between functional and experiential health and that within the social determination of experiential health itself. In conclusion, then, "health" in a capitalist society is nothing more than the prevailing standoff at a point in time between its functional and experiential aspects, between the tendency for the accumulation process to reduce its subsumed human populations to the status of resources employed for its expansion and the tendency of people to seek their own transcendent (of the accumulation process) fulfillment. To be sure, the parameters of this standoff can be expected to vary from society to society, within societies over time, and across age, sex, race, and class differences. This dialectical development of the definition of health will be elaborated historically in the second part of this article.

In sum, the attempt has been made here to chart the paradigmatic development of notions of "health." In Western culture the first, and still most prominent, paradigm is that of the machine model of the body and the germ theory of disease. Because of its inability to incorporate emotional and psychosomatic processes, and the social, rather than individual, causes of illness into its paradigm, it yields logically to the social epidemiology paradigm. Both, however, are limited in their capacity to generate a notion of organismic integrity, i.e. "health," since both view "health" as independent of the form of society in which it is studied. Given contemporary practices concerning stress, cancer, and other environmentally induced illnesses, "health" is something other than the lack of organismic breakdown, the definition implied by both of these paradigms. Instead, a functional dimension must be recognized as part and parcel of a definition of health which purports to describe accurately health behavior in contemporary capitalist society. After an analytic discussion of the social and economic dynamics of capitalist society, it was concluded that an appropriate definition of health must recognize the inherent contradictions, in such a society, between functional and experiential health, on the one hand, and within the social determination of experiential health itself, on the other. In the remaining two sections of part one, this dialectical view of the definition of health will be compared with other existing definitions of health, and the possibilities of a normative definition of health will be considered.

Critical Review of Existing Definitions of Health

The above discussion of health can be usefully amplified by considering contemporary definitions of health. Perhaps the most widely known is that of the World Health Organization: ". . . a complete state of physical, mental, and social well being, not merely the absence of disease . . . ." Similar, though not identical, is that of Rossdale: "the product of a harmonized relationship between man and his ecology" (6). Both tend to be utopian definitions in expressing what "health" ought to be, but differ in that the former is defined in terms of outcome, whereas the latter is defined in terms of structure and process. Neither, however, incorporates the structural limitations to its attainment inherent in capitalist society, and hence, neither accurately depicts health behavior in *contemporary* society. Rossdale's discussion (6) clearly recognizes many of these limitations, however.

Along similar lines, but in nonutopian terms, Dubos offers the following: "a modus vivendi enabling imperfect men to achieve a rewarding and not too painful existence while they cope with an imperfect world" (29, p. 67). There are several difficulties with this definition, even on its own terms. First, it is ahistorical in the sense of not indicating the (possibly alienating or alienated) terms on which existence is "rewarding." Second, it is not clear how Dubos' definition of "health" differs from "wealth" or many other things.

Turning from experiential definitions to more functionally oriented definitions, perhaps the most renowned is that of Parsons: "the state of optimum *capacity* of an individual for the effective performance of the roles and tasks for which he has been socialized" (12, p. 117). In this definition it appears that the ability to perform is the sole requisite of "health," and that any experience of illness does not, in itself, mitigate the achievement of "health" in Parsonian terms. More specifically, if the performance of one's work is itself pathogenic (coal mining, asbestos processing, textile manufacturing, etc.), Parsons' definition identifies the result as illness only when it results in the absence from work, or, more generally, the incapacity to perform as "socialized." Furthermore, since there are no limitations on Parsons' use of the category of role socialization, the possibilities for alienation in the present circumstances leave the normative pretense of the definition somewhat minimal. Still, there is a further difficulty, even within Parsons' functional orientation, namely, that it suffers from a particular form of ahistoricism. In capitalist society, functional health, subordinated as it is to the process of accumulation, refers only to the capacity to contribute to that process, not the capacity to perform any role or task, productive or not, as implied by Parsons' definition.

Dreitzel (30, p. xi) resolves this point by arguing that "health is institutionally defined as the capability to help produce the very surplus the owners of the means of production appropriate." Although this is a clear and consistent statement of what has been argued as functional "health," it suffers in its economic determinism in not recognizing the dialectical nature of "health" and the very political experiential dimension of it.

Finally, though it is not concerned with definitions of health per se, the increasing tendency for neoclassical economists to view health as human capital (earning capacity) deserves some comment. The human capital school developed in the early 1950s at a time when economists began investigating the sources of economic growth. From this came the realization that not only the quantity of resources employed but also their quality were central to an understanding of the rate of economic growth. Specifically singled out was the quality of labor resources with a focus on the amount of embodied education, job training, and health care. Expenditures for these labor quality-enhancing services came to be known as investments in human capital, and increasingly the rates of return to these investments are analyzed in terms of their contributions to economic growth and to individual earning capacity (31, 32), which amount to much the same thing.

What is significant about this development in economics is that it tends to lend ideological support to the notion of "health" as functional to the accumulation process and will likely become the analytical basis for policy determination of the appropriate level of expenditure in health care.

Toward a Normative Conception of "Health"

Beginning with the premise that "health" in contemporary society is the prevailing contradiction between its experiential and functional dimensions, a normative conception of "health" could be defined as a situation in which the two are "in equilibrium," that is, a situation in which for a given individual the experience of well-being coincides with the ability to fulfil his or her social role. Attractive as this construction may at first appear, it is ahistorical and, as such, indeterminate. This can be seen by considering two polar types of societies. First, in an unalienated, unobjectified society (socialism, as defined above), it is at least theoretically possible that the equilibrium defined above is possible, and in this case it would appear to have substantial normative significance. The equilibrium is also possible, however, in a highly totalitarian society in which psychological and physiological mechanisms of social control are widely used, one in which well-being is defined *as* the ability to perform as socialized. (And the increasingly significant use of "ethical" psychoactive and antihypertensive drugs, psychosurgery, and adjustment-oriented psychotherapy in our own society would appear to be a move in this latter direction.) In this (totalitarian) case, little normative significance is evident, since experiential "health," itself, is highly alienated.

Analytically it would appear that the transcendent, normative quest for the resolution of the dialectic of "health" must be based in a mode of analysis that is explicitly historical and that seeks the social conditions necessary for the liberation of experience from objectification. Concretely, the resolution will be based in a mode of social organization that renders these conditions possible.

APPLICATION OF THE THEORY

For whatever reasons that healing as an activity (not necessarily as a profession) originated anthropologically in primitive societies, inevitably it came to play a larger social role as it became incorporated into the social (largely religious) patterns, symbols, and metaphors (7, 33, 34, pp. 2-4). To the present day there has always been an intensive interplay between "advances" in curing and their circumscription by the larger patterns and symbols of the society. In other words, the functional aspects of "health" arise historically out of the incorporation of curing into the larger ritual structure of the society. The teasing apart of the functional and experiential aspects of "health," therefore, becomes a rather delicate and complex exercise.

The Enlightenment period (18th century) in Europe fostered both the advance and the compromise of "health." Most importantly, it formed the basis of the secularization of thought, particularly the sanctuary for science and its applications. As a consequence, science was seen as, and indeed became, a mechanism for improving human (experiential) health and welfare (34, p. 22). In supplanting medieval religious metaphors about disease, however, the Enlightenment also provided for their secular replacements. In the case of the human body, the new metaphor was the machine (Descartes). Early medical scientists such as Vesalius and Harvey saw the body merely as the *homologue* of the machine, i.e. structured similarly. With the growth of mercantilism and the mercantilist state, together with their military and strategic implications, the human body came also to be seen as the *analogue* of the machine, i.e. functioning (purposively) similarly.

As Broekman has argued:

> It is of considerable importance for the sociology of knowledge that it was precisely during the time of change in the attitude towards one's own corporality under the influence of emerging industrial norms that the problem of having-a-body and being-a-body was rethought in the context of Philosophical Anthropology (Husserl, Plessner, Marcel, Sartre). The fact that the mode of having-a-body has generally come to prevail indicates a major shift of norms. Only on the basis of this mode is one open to the experience of being-a-body. We call this an instrumental attitude toward the body. The body becomes one's own body by reflection upon the *function* of the body (35).

Moreover, Rosen suggests:

> Taking as a point of departure the mercantilist position in relation to health, a few farseeing men had been led in the seventeenth century to adumbrate the idea of health as a significant element of national policy. Problems of health were considered chiefly in connection with the aim of maintaining and augmenting a healthy population and thus in terms of their significance for the political and economic strength of the state. On a theoretical plane, this idea had been developed in varying degree in different countries.

> However, owing to the lack of knowledge and administrative machinery, it had nowhere been possible to develop and to implement a health policy on a national basis . . . until the later nineteenth century (34, p. 19).

The rise of science in the mercantilist period set the stage, then, for the simultaneous emancipation and objectification of the human organism. Given the subordination of science to the larger society, "health" became significantly subordinated to the mercantilist state and later to production itself. This is true not only of somatic concerns, but mental as well (36).

"Health" in America

Applying this general discussion of "health" to a specific country—the United States—is revealing. Beginning in the 17th century, American society was organized almost entirely into self-sufficient, but not unrepressive, village life, with agriculture and artisanship the primary economic activities. By the mid-18th century, there was, in both secular and religious terms, a growing ideology of independence, self-sufficiency, equality (before God and the law), and anti-mercantilism. This growing ideology, together with the increasingly repressive mercantilism of Great Britain, produced the American Revolution. Thus came solidification of the American state, an emerging American capitalism (Hamiltonianism), and the growth of cities with a nascent urban manufacture. In reaction to these came Shay's Rebellion and a second "Great Awakening" that reasserted human equality before God, now strengthened by a corresponding equality before the law institutionalized by the U.S. Constitution. These in turn led to the period of Jacksonianism: the rise of the common man and individualism in the second quarter of the 19th century.

Out of these cultural developments grew new departures in medicine. Along with the eclectic and folk practices in existence throughout this period, two new practices of medicine emerged by the 1840s: the Popular Health Movement and Thomsonianism. Both stressed self-reliance, self-help, prevention, and whole-person treatment. As such, they both encouraged and reinforced a relatively unalienated form of experiential "health."

In contrast, scientific medicine was a strictly imported commodity. Virtually all scientific physicians practicing in the U.S. before 1890 were educated in Europe, and that form of practice remained a rather small portion of medical practice until the end of the 19th century.

Given the largely agricultural nature of American society prior to the Civil War, however, functional "health" was largely nonoperational for the white population. The most systematic expression of functional "health" in 19th-century America, and possibly to the present, was found on the ante-bellum southern plantations.

For slaves in the ante-bellum South, to whom health care was far more systematically available and for whom health status indicators were significantly superior to those of freed blacks and poor whites in the North and South (37), health care was strictly an investment, or more accurately, a maintenance expenditure (38, pp. 279-321). Physicians provided prepaid contracts to slaveholders to cover the cost of caring for the slaves, and an entire holding of slaves would often be moved to a more healthy location in times of epidemic, even at the cost of a whole year's production. Irish laborers were sometimes hired in order to save the slaves from working in malaria-infested areas. However, medical care was withheld from slaves when the anticipated cost (times the probability of failure) did not seem justified in the eyes of the slaveholder (39).

Because slaves were literally administered as means of production, it is understandable that their mortality rates were lower than those of freed blacks and lower class whites. As they represented real capital holdings of the slaveholders, those holders had, together with the paternalism of their plantation administration, a clear economic interest in seeing to the maintenance of that property (insofar as it did not exceed the replacement cost or capital value), whereas there were no similar incentives to extend health care to lower class whites.

With the end of the Civil War came the Age of the Robber Barons, full-scale industrialization, the concentration of industry, the legalization of the joint stock company (corporation), and the consolidation of power by the leading industrialists, which was most clearly visible in the 1890s. This consolidation took the forms of municipal reform, centralization and standardization of schools, and scientific management of industry. Through a series of Carnegie Foundation-sponsored studies, professional education was transformed from apprenticeship to university training, thereby upgrading the class origins of the practitioners of those professions.

One such Carnegie-sponsored study was the Flexner Report which effectively made illegal all practices of medicine other than the allopathic form. Having gained the monopoly over the legitimate practice of medicine, scientific-oriented physicians proceeded to redefine illness clinically rather than experientially. In addition, they deemphasized prevention and self-help, relegated women's normal health behavior such as childbirth to the category of illness, suppressed midwifery, and, as a result, substantially alienated experiential "health." And thus it remained until the 1960s.

Functional "health" has not yet become the systematic basis of national health policy, although increasingly throughout the 20th century indications of its desirability have begun to surface in corporate circles. For example, in writing the introduction to his text on occupational medicine in 1925, J.D. Hackett stated:

> Chickens, race-horses, and circus monkeys are fed, housed, trained, and kept up to the highest physical pitch in order to secure a full return from them as producers in their respective functions. The same principle applies to human beings; increased production cannot be expected from workers unless some attention is paid to their physical environment and needs.
> The object of this book is to show those who manage plants and are, therefore, responsible for the management of medical departments, how the workers' health may be maintained and improved as a means of increasing production.
> ... [they] must be able to guide and direct the medical staff just as [they guide] other technical branches of plant operation (40, p. iii).

Similarly, in reporting to President Truman in 1949 concerning conditions in the strike-bound steel industry, the Steel Industry Board stated in part that:

> Social insurance and pensions should be considered a part of normal business costs to take care of temporary and permanent depreciation in the human "machine" in much the same way as provision is made for depreciation and insurance of plant and machinery. This obligation should be among the first charges on revenues (41, p. 8).

With the advent of the late 1950s and continuing throughout the 1960s began a full decade of social activism. Starting with the lower class civil rights and anti-poverty movements, this activity moved into middle class circles, particularly the young, with the anti-war, women's liberation, and anti-corruption movements. Out of this ferment has grown a renewed popular interest in matters related to health. Widespread personal efforts and interests have developed in the areas of diet, health food, anti-smoking, exercises, the deprofessionalization of medicine (particularly by women), and the struggle against occupational disease and injury. Hence, the alienating nature of contemporary scientific medicine has come under attack at virtually the same time that its delivery capability is widely recognized as being in a state of "crisis" (42).

Today, many conflicting strategies for resolution of the contradictions in the fee-for-service delivery system are being promoted, but virtually no attention is being paid to the methodological focus of medicine itself. A growing number of major corporations are pursuing the idea of reestablishing the delivery system in employer-sponsored health maintenance organizations through the expansion of their existing occupational medical departments. On a micro-level this promises, through the equation of the company with the family doctor, to institutionalize a system of medicine not unlike that practiced in the plantation South.

On a macro-level, particularly given the difficulties in the larger American economy, there may be a tendency to rationalize the aggregate expenditures in health care through the calculus of investment in human capital. This would intensify the health pressure on those elements in the population not central to or easily replaceable in the process of capital accumulation. More generally, this would tend to retard the advances in experiential "health" of the 1960s. Perhaps even more important, functional "health" would for the first time in American history move to center stage in the execution of national health policy.

Yet such corporate-sponsored "reforms" would be quite successful in eliminating most of the strictly structural defects in the contemporary American health care system. They would eliminate the duplicated services, unnecessary surgery, fragmented specialties, unnecessary hospital construction and utilization, and perhaps, the runaway inflation inherent in the system today.

Without a clear focus on "health," health care analysts will miss the pernicious implications of the corporate-sponsored reforms, and will, indeed, become unconscious ideological supporters for that pattern of reform. A strictly technical orientation to the analysis of health care reform is not sufficient: "health" itself must be the basis by which reforms are judged progressive or retrogressive.

Acknowledgments—The development of this article has benefitted substantially from the comments, criticisms, and suggestions of a very large number of people. Unfortunately, not all of them could be incorporated into this version and, no doubt, it is the worse for that lack. Nonetheless, I would like to personally thank Roger Battistella, Howard Berliner, Erwin Blackstone, Michael Clark, John Condry, Sarah Elbert, Joe Eyer, John Ford, Tor Holm, Vicente Navarro, Ulrich Neisser, Jonathan Reader, Jack Salmon, George Silver, and Karl Weick. The responsibility for errors and imprecisions which remain accrue to the author.

REFERENCES

1. Kuhn, T. *The Structure of Scientific Revolutions.* University of Chicago Press, Chicago, 1962.
2. Ginsburg, H., and Opper, S. *Piaget's Theory of Intellectual Development: An Introduction.* Prentice-Hall, Englewood Cliffs, N.J., 1969.

3. Neisser, U. *Cognition and Reality*, Ch. IV, p. 26. Freeman, San Francisco, in press.
4. Luria, A. Towards the problem of the historical nature of psychological processes. *International Journal of Psychology* 6(4):259-272, 1971.
5. Berry, J. W. Radical cultural relativism and the concept of intelligence. In *Mental Tests and Cultural Adaptation*, edited by L. J. Cronbach and P. J. Drenth, pp. 77-88. Humanities Press, New York, 1972.
6. Rossdale, M. Health in a sick society. *New Left Review* No. 34, 82-90, 1965.
7. Levi-Stauss, C. *Structural Anthropology*, Ch. IX. Basic Books, New York, 1963.
8. Romøren, T. I. Body-medicine-society: Some comments concerning the ideology of somatic medicine. In *Helse i Norge*, edited by T. I. Romøren. Pax, Oslo, 1973 (unpublished translation by Knut Ringen, Johns Hopkins University School of Hygiene and Public Health).
9. Eyer, J. Hypertension as a disease of modern society. *Int. J. Health Serv.* 5(4):539-558, 1975.
10. Bernstein, P. J. Carcinogens. *Boston Sunday Globe*, p. A-4. January 19, 1975.
11. Fromm, E. *The Sane Society*. Fawcett, Greenwich, Conn., 1955.
12. Parsons, T. In *Patients, Physicians, and Illness*, edited by E. Gartly Jaco, Ed. 2, pp. 107-127. Free Press, New York, 1972.
13. Baran, P., and Hobsbawm, E. The method of historical materialism. In *The Capitalist System*, edited by R. Edwards, M. Reich, and T. Weisskopf, pp. 53-56. Prentice-Hall, Englewood Cliffs, N.J., 1972.
14. Brodeur, P. *Expendable Americans*. Viking Press, New York, 1974.
15. O'Brien, M.-W., and Page, J. A. *Bitter Wages: Ralph Nader's Study Group Report on Disease and Injury on the Job*. Grossman, New York, 1973.
16. Kelman, S. Book Review of *The Rising Cost of Hospital Care* by M. Feldstein. *Int. J. Health Serv.* 3(2):311-314, 1973.
17. Whyte, W. H. *The Organization Man*. Simon & Schuster, New York, 1956.
18. Bowles, S. Unequal education and the reproduction of the hierarchical division of labor. In *The Capitalist System*, edited by R. Edwards, M. Reich, and T. Weisskopf, pp. 218-229. Prentice-Hall, Englewood Cliffs, N.J., 1972.
19. Katz, M. *The Irony of Early School Reform*. Harvard University Press, Cambridge, 1968.
20. Spring, J. *Education and the Rise of the Corporate State*. Beacon, Boston, 1972.
21. Katz, M. *Class Bureaucracy and Schools: The Illusion of Educational Change in America*. Praeger, New York, 1971.
22. Tyack, D. *One Best System: A History of American Urban Education*. Harvard University Press, Cambridge, 1975.
23. Henry, J. *Culture against Man*. Vintage, New York, 1965.
24. Laing, R. D. *The Politics of Experience*. Pantheon, New York, 1967.
25. Breggin, P. New information in the debate over psychosurgery. *Congressional Record* 92nd Congress, second session: E3380-E3386, March 30, 1972.
26. Marcuse, H. *One-Dimensional Man*. Beacon Press, Boston, 1964.
27. Task Force Report to the Secretary of the U.S. Department of Health, Education, and Welfare. *Work in America*. Massachusetts Institute of Technology Press, Cambridge, 1973.
28. Marx, K. *The Eighteenth Brumaire of Louis Bonaparte*. International Publishers, New York, 1963.
29. Dubos, R. *Medicine, Man, and Environment*. Praeger, New York, 1968.
30. Dreitzel, H. P. In *The Social Organization of Health*, edited by H. P. Dreitzel, pp. v-xvii. Macmillan, New York, 1971.
31. Special issue on "Investment in Human Beings." *Journal of Political Economy* 70(5, Part 2), 1962.
32. Grossman, M. On the concept of health capital and the demand for health. *Journal of Political Economy* 80(2):223-255, 1972.
33. Turner, V. *The Forest of Symbols: Aspects of Ndembu Ritual*. Cornell University Press, Ithaca, N.Y., 1970.
34. Rosen, G. In *The Hospital in Modern Society*, edited by E. Freidson, pp. 1-36. Free Press, Glencoe, 1963.
35. Broekman, J. M. Quoted in and translated by Dreitzel, H. P. in *The Social Organization of Health*, pp. ix-x. Macmillan, New York, 1971.
36. Foucault, M. *Madness and Civilization: A History of Insanity in the Age of Reason*. Pantheon, New York, 1971.
37. Postell, W. D. *The Health of Slaves on Southern Plantations*. Louisiana State University Press, Baton Rouge, 1961.
38. Stampp, K. M. *The Peculiar Institution*. Knopf, New York, 1956.
39. Shryock, R. H. Medicine in the old south. In *Medicine in America: Historical Essays*, edited by R. H. Shryock. Johns Hopkins Press, Baltimore, 1966.

40. Hackett, J. D. *Health Maintenance in Industry,* Shaw, Chicago, 1925.
41. *Report to the President of the United States on the Labor Dispute in the Basic Steel Industry.* Steel Industry Board, Washington, D.C., September 10, 1949.
42. Special issue of *Fortune,* January 1970.

CHAPTER 2

Functionalism and After?
Theory and Developments
in Social Science
Applied to the Health Field

Ronald Frankenberg

Social concern with health and medical care does not begin with sociology. Indeed, it is possible to argue that this is where it ends. A theoretical concern with the social prerequisites of health and disease might begin in prehistory or in the antiquity of Galen or Hippocrates. Like much else in sociology, it should at least start with Marx. I shall argue that the insights and approaches of Marx, Sigerist, and Shaw are characteristically emasculated by Parsons and his successors. Even the partial victory of sociology in the medical school has been pyrrhic; it has succumbed to repressive tolerance at the cost of its bite. This should not surprise us since sociology humanizing medicine is the blind leading the blind. Both suffer from the same theoretical difficulty to which the most successful of modern applied sociologists of medicine has drawn our attention, namely the failure to realize that the universality of contradiction lies in its particularity.

Let me explain myself. The doctor is presented in clinical practice with a series of individuals; to universalize his treatment he must theorize—he must adopt a policy of classification of patients, symptoms, or diseases, or a combination of the three. Foucault (1) has shown us how this theory has changed through the centuries, but for the given doctor it has usually been implicit rather than stated. The consequence has been for both individual, at any one moment of time, and the mass historically, a veering from external to internal, from organic to psychologic, from vitalistic to mechanistic, explanation.

The insoluble problem which has bedevilled the healer is the relationship between the individual exemplar and the mass. To understand this, it is necessary to see a systematic relationship between the part and the whole. It is at this point that the sociologist has sought to help, but alas it is at precisely this problem that the sociologist himself has come to a halt. I shall argue that in neither case is this accidental, for both sociologist and doctor it would if they passed this point be suicidal—the sociologist would become an intelligent historian and the doctor a human being rather than a professional demigod. Furthermore, both would be potential revolutionaries.

MARX'S *CAPITAL* AS KEY TO MEDICAL SOCIOLOGY

The clue (as to much else) lies in Marx's *Capital* (2). Here he describes in simultaneously abstract theoretical and empirical observational terms medical conditions in particular places and times. He relates these to conditions of work themselves historically determined not just by the historical accident of a particular period but by the nature of the social relations within it. For later comparison it is necessary to give this theory here, albeit in highly condensed form. Marx argued that the nature of all social relationships within any epoch of history was largely determined by the nature of production relations. Particularly, it depended on the fate and mode of appropriation of the surplus to his needs that a man was capable of producing. Within the capitalist system where "free" men "freely" offered their services to an employer, surplus value was acquired by buying the *time* of a worker at its value: what it cost to produce it. This cost was the cost of maintaining a man at work—food, clothing, and shelter for him, as well as for his family—since it was necessary that he remain at work in perpetuity. For various reasons which I need not enter into here, it was necessary in order for the capitalist to maintain his profit (let alone make it greater) to increase this surplus value. This could be achieved either by making the men produce more—through working harder, through longer hours, through machinery—or by reducing the cost of the man's time—by cheapening the element "needed" to keep him alive, or by employing his family.[1] Marx explores the interrelated consequences of the pressure to increase surplus value on relations within the family, on nutrition, on rest, on morals and the relationships of the sexes, on the general physical characteristics of the population, and on the prevalence of industrial diseases. I confine myself to two examples. The first is derived from the district in which the University of Keele is now situated (2, pp. 229-230):

> Dr. Greenhow states that the average duration of life in the pottery districts of Stoke-on-Trent and Wolstanton is extraordinarily short. Although in the district of Stoke, only 36.6% and in Wolstanton only 30.4% of the adult male population above 20 are employed in the potteries, among the men of that age in the first district more than half, in the second, nearly two-fifths of the whole deaths are the result of pulmonary diseases among the potters. Dr. Boothroyd, a medical practitioner at Hanley, says: "Each successive generation of potters is more dwarfed and less robust than the preceding one." In like manner another doctor, Mr. M'Bean: "Since he began to practise among the potters 25 years ago, he had observed a marked degeneration especially shown in diminution of stature and breadth." These statements are taken from the report of Dr. Greenhow in 1860.
>
> From the report of the Commissioners in 1863, the following: Dr. J. T. Arledge, senior physician of the North Staffordshire Infirmary, says: "The potters as a class, both men and women, represent a degenerated population, both physically and morally. They are, as a rule, stunted in growth, ill-shaped, and frequently ill-formed in the chest; they become prematurely old, and are certainly short-lived; they are phlegmatic and

---

[1] Lenin (3) gives a nice example of the simultaneous use of both methods in Russia. The increasing growth of potatoes for the manufacture of alcohol from starch as capitalist-organized factories spread into the countryside simultaneously lowered the cost of feeding the workers by substituting bread with potatoes. We can only guess at the health cost of this, as we can guess at the change produced by the substitution noted by Cobbett in 18th-century England of potatoes and weak tea for bread, beef, and ale. Whether it is an advantage to be able to measure accurately the similar effects of the simultaneous introduction of cash crop tobacco or coffee and low-protein cassava in modern Africa remains to be seen.

bloodless, and exhibit their debility of constitution by obstinate attacks of dyspepsia, and disorders of the liver and kidneys, and by rheumatism. But of all diseases they are especially prone to chest-disease, to pneumonia, phthisis, bronchitis, and asthma. One form would appear peculiar to them, and is known as potter's asthma, or potter's consumption. Scrofula attacking the glands, or bones, or other parts of the body, is a disease of two-thirds or more of the potters. . . . That the 'degenerescence' of the population of this district is not even greater than it is, is due to the constant recruiting from the adjacent country, and intermarriages with more healthy races."

Mr. Charles Parsons, late house surgeon of the same institution, writes in a letter to Commissioner Longe, amongst other things: "I can only speak from personal observation and not from statistical data, but I do not hesitate to assert that my indignation has been aroused again and again at the sight of poor children whose health has been sacrificed to gratify the avarice of either parents or employers." He enumerates the causes of the diseases of the potters, and sums them up in the phrase, "long hours."

Another example of Marx's own words (2, pp. 238-241):

From the motley crowd of labourers of all callings, ages, sexes, that press on us more busily than the souls of the slain on Ulysses, on whom—without referring to the blue books under their arms—we see at a glance the mark of over-work, let us take two more figures whose striking contrast proves that before capital all men are alike—a milliner and a blacksmith.

In the last week of June, 1863, all the London daily papers published a paragraph with the "sensational" heading, "Death from simple over-work." It dealt with the death of the milliner, Mary Anne Walkley, 20 years of age, employed in a highly respectable dressmaking establishment, exploited by a lady with the pleasant name of Elise. The old, often-told story, was once more recounted. This girl worked, on an average, 16½ hours, during the season often 30 hours, without a break, whilst her failing labour-power was revived by occasional supplies of sherry, port or coffee. It was just now the height of the season. It was necessary to conjure up in the twinkling of an eye the gorgeous dresses for the noble ladies bidden to the ball in honour of the newly imported Princess of Wales. Mary Anne Walkley had worked without intermission for 26½ hours, with 60 other girls, 30 in one room, that only afforded one-third of the cubic feet of air required for them. At night, they slept in pairs in one of the stifling holes into which the bedroom was divided by partitions of board. And this was one of the best millinery establishments in London. Mary Anne Walkley fell ill on the Friday, died on Sunday, without, to the astonishment of Madame Elise, having previously completed the work in hand. The doctor, Mr. Keys, called too late to the death-bed, duly bore witness before the coroner's jury that "Mary Anne Walkley had died from long hours of work in an over-crowded workroom, and a too small and badly-ventilated bedroom." In order to give the doctor a lesson in good manners, the coroner's jury thereupon brought in a verdict that "the deceased had died of apoplexy, but there was reason to fear that her death had been accelerated by over-work in an over-crowded workroom. . . ." "Our white slaves," cried the *Morning Star*, the organ of the free-traders, Cobden and Bright, "our white slaves, who are toiled into the grave, for the most part silently pine and die."

It is not in dressmakers' rooms that working to death is the order of the day, but in a thousand other places; in every place I had almost said, where a "thriving business" has to be done. . . . We will take the blacksmith as a type. If the poets were true, there is no man so hearty, so merry, as the blacksmith; he rises early and strikes his sparks before the sun; he eats and drinks and sleeps as no other man. Working in moderation, he is, in fact, in one of the best of human positions, physically speaking. But we follow him into the city or town, and we see the stress of work on that strong man, and what then is his position in the death-rate of 31 per thousand per annum, or 11 above the mean of the male adults of the country in its entirety. The occupation, instinctive almost as a portion of human art, unobjectionable as a branch of human industry, is made by mere excess of work, the destroyer of the man. He can strike so many blows, to walk so many more steps, to breathe so many more breaths per day, and to increase altogether a fourth of his life. He meets the effort; the result is, that producing for a limited time a fourth more work, he dies at 37 for 50.

Finally, I would like to quote from Marx another passage (2, pp. 395-396) where the ill health recorded is not directly industrial disease.

We have already alluded to the physical deterioration as well of the children and young persons as of the women, whom machinery, first directly in the factories that shoot up on its basis, and then indirectly in all the remaining branches of industry, subjects to the exploitation of capital. In this place, therefore, we dwell only on one point, the enormous mortality, during the first few years of their life, of the children of the operatives. In sixteen of the registration districts into which England is divided, there are, for every 100,000 children alive under the age of one year, only 9000 deaths in a year on an average (in one district only 7047): in 24 districts the deaths are over 12,000; in 48 districts over 12,000, but under 13,000; in 22 districts over 20,000; in 25 districts over 21,000; in 17 over 22,000; in 11 over 23,000; in Hoo, Wolverhampton, Ashton-under-Lyme, and Preston, over 24,000; in Nottingham, Stockport, and Bradford, over 25,000; in Wisbeach, 26,000; and in Manchester 26,126. As was shown by an official medical inquiry in the year 1861, the high death-rates are, apart from local causes, principally due to the employment of the mothers away from their homes, and to the neglect and maltreatment consequent on her absence, such as, amongst others, insufficient nourishment, unsuitable food, and dosing with opiates; besides this, there arises an unnatural estrangement between mother and child, and as a consequence intentional starving and poisoning of the children. In those agricultural districts, "where a minimum in the employment of women exists, the death-rate is on the other hand very low." The inquiry-Commission of 1861 led, however, to the unexpected result, that in some purely agricultural districts bordering on the North Sea, the death-rate of children under one year old almost equalled that of the worst factory districts. Dr. Julian Hunter was therefore commissioned to investigate this phenomenon on the spot. His report is incorporated with the "Sixth Report on Public Health." Up to that time it was supposed, that the children were decimated by malaria, and other diseases peculiar to low-lying and marshy districts. But the inquiry showed the very opposite, namely, that the same cause which drove away malaria, the conversion of the land, from a morass in winter and a scanty pasture in summer, into fruitful corn land, created the exceptional death-rate of the infants. The 70 medical men, whom Dr. Hunter examined in that district, were "wonderfully in accord" on this point. In fact, the revolution in the mode of cultivation had led to the introduction of the industrial system. Married women, who work in gangs along with boys and girls, are, for a stipulated sum of money, placed at the disposal of the farmer, by a man called the "undertaker," who contracts for the whole gang. "These gangs will sometimes travel many miles from their own village; they are to be met morning and evening on the roads, dressed in short petticoats with suitable coats and boots, and sometimes trousers, looking wonderfully strong and healthy, but tainted with a customary immorality, and heedless of the fatal results which their love of this busy and independent life is bringing on their unfortunate offspring who are pining at home." Every phenomenon of the factory districts is here reproduced, including, but to a greater extent, ill-disguised infanticide, and dosing children with opiates. "My knowledge of such evils," says Dr. Simon, the medical officer of the Privy Council and editor in chief of the Reports on Public Health, "may excuse the profound misgiving with which I regard any large industrial employment of adult women."

This passage carried the interesting (and topical) footnote (2, p. 396):

In the agricultural as well as in the factory districts the consumption of opium among the grown-up labourers, both male and female, is extending daily. "To push the sale of opiate . . . is the great aim of some enterprising wholesale merchants. By druggists it is considered the leading article." Infants that take opiates "shrank up into little old men," or "wizzened like little monkeys." We here see how India and China avenged themselves on England.

I do not quote these passages to endorse John Simon's profound misgivings about the industrial employment of adult women, or for local color. The point I wish to make is that they are embedded within a theory of social change which is historically situated, and the remedy for the evils described is seen by Marx not as the impracticable palliative of Simon (stop women working) but as fundamental social change. Does the development of more modern and effective palliatives justify a more empiricist, accepting sociology of medicine?

THE CONTRIBUTION OF HENRY SIGERIST: LABOR POWER AND HEALTH

A natural link between Marx and the modern writer is Henry Sigerist (4, 5) whose work *Socialised Medicine in the Soviet Union* (1937) (4), although basically like the Webb's one of Fabian enthusiasm, also begins with a summary of Marx's theory of capitalism.

In his lecture "The Place of the Physician in Modern Society" given in 1946, Sigerist (5) makes his fundamental assumptions clear. First, as in all his writing, he places modern medicine within an historical context. He quotes with approval (5, p. 69) a 19th-century German author who had

> ... pointed out that the state had as one of its purposes the protection of the people's property, that the majority of people, however, had only one possession, their labor power, one which was entirely determined by their health. He therefore concluded that the state had the duty to protect the people's health as their most valuable property. If the purpose of the state is to promote the general welfare of the people, then there can be no doubt that the protection of health must be one of the primary concerns of government.
>
> [He continues to argue:] Medicine, usually regarded as a natural science, actually is a social science because its goal is social. *Its primary target must be to keep individuals adjusted to their environment as useful members of society, or to readjust them when they have dropped out* as a result of illness [emphasis added].

Thus we see that Sigerist is already viewing medicine in functionalist, conservative terms in relation to society. His enthusiasm for the Soviet Union (like that of Sydney Webb and Bernard Shaw) seemed more paradoxical then than it does now. He is a radical reformist rather than a revolutionary. Radical reformism, even placed firmly within an historical context, especially when linked with an elitist view of the function of the profession, is synonymous with intelligent conservatism. This led Sigerist to see the medical function as fourfold: The first charge upon physicians is the promotion of health through education in the school and outside, and especially through physical education and exercise. By getting his patients to stand on their heads, he stands Marx on his (5, p. 70):

> Labor power spent in the process of production must be restored. Periods of work must be followed by periods of rest, and this rest should in certain cases be under medical supervision. In handling our automobiles we have learned that it is cheaper to have them overhauled periodically and to have minor repairs made before the car breaks down. A program of human conservation would make use of the same principle. The promotion of health moreover requires the provision of a decent standard of living with the best possible living and labor conditions. The promotion of the people's health is undoubtedly an eminently social task that calls for the coordinated efforts of large groups, of the statesman, labor, industry, of the educator, and of the physician who, as an expert in matters of health, must define norms and set standards.

The second charge Sigerist enjoined upon physicians is the prevention of disease, especially for groups at risk (5, p. 71):

> Especially menaced for physiological reasons are women in pregnancy, childbirth, and childbed, infants, young children, and aged people. Socially threatened as a result of their occupation are industrial workers. Society, therefore, called upon the doctor to develop special methods and institutions for the protection of mother and child, for the care of the aged, and for the protection of labor.

The third charge, to be entered into when the first two have in individual cases inevitably failed, is the restoration of health, and this too is seen by Sigerist in a social context (5, p. 71):

> In taking the history of a patient, the physician endeavors to obtain a picture of his living and working conditions, of his relationships to the family and other social groups, because the illness may have been caused directly or indirectly by a wrong mode of living or by social maladjustment. The doctor is an individual, to be sure, but is at the same time also a member of society who, in the patient, treats another individual who is also a member of a group. Treatment may consist in the correction of a social relationship.

Finally, in Sigerist's view, the physician must be concerned with social rehabilitation: getting the worker back to work, and the mother back to the family. Sigerist mentions in passing other roles of the physician in relation to the state, as in the legal system—"the administration of justice would be impossible without his services" (5, p. 72)—and in giving advice on poverty and housing programs, and ends his brief survey (5, p. 74):

> We see him [the physician in modern society] as a scientist, educator, and social worker, ready to cooperate in teamwork, in close touch with the people he disinterestedly serves, a friend and leader who directs all his efforts toward the promotion of health and prevention of disease and becomes a therapist when his previous efforts have broken down—the social physician protecting the people and guiding them to a healthier and happier life.

Sigerist as a Conservative

This view is sharply opposed to the conservatism of the American Medical Association, and its elitism is neatly and unconsciously disguised by its humanism. It is in accord with the medical system of the Soviet Union as seen through Fabian eyes in the thirties, and with the National Health Service of Britain in the fifties. In contrast to its successors, Sigerist's elitism was placed in historical context. Until the rise of the Chinese non-specialist barefoot "doctors," black power, Puerto Rican rebellion, and women's liberation (6), there had not been any challenge to medical elitism in social practice. It is not surprising therefore, considering sociologists' lack of general education in literature and history, that they should not see its fallacies and dangers until woken to them partially by Wootton (7), but mainly by Freidson (8) and Zola (9).

GEORGE BERNARD SHAW'S NEGLECTED VIEWS

As Boxill (10) has pointed out, however, one writer, schooled significantly in practice by working in a local authority, challenged most of the elements of the picture. He was, of course, another Fabian—George Bernard Shaw. Boxill emphasizes Shaw's vitalist philosophy. My concern is rather with the social bases of Shaw's thinking, and his criticism of medicine because it sees itself as a profession, while to Shaw it is both a capitalist device and an elitist concept. Although Shaw's view on and analysis of medicine are most popularly known from his play *The Doctor's Dilemma* (11) and the preface to it, together with the relevant passages in *Everybody's Political What's What* (12), he published a series of articles in *The English Review* in 1918 and reprinted them in the book *Doctors' Delusions* in 1932 (13). I have used Boxill's summaries of the last.

Shaw Sees Medicine Whole and in Context

The significance of his criticism is in its systematic nature: the medical profession is seen in historical and social context, a part of the whole.

It emerges most clearly in his prescription for a national health service. He starts by contrasting the treatment of Hahnemann (the inventor of homeopathy) and Jenner (the alleged deviser of vaccination). Both apply the same principle; the one is reviled, the other a hero. Why? Shaw seeks an answer in the total context of medicine as a trade. The former represents a threat to trade interests; the latter laid the base for a large industry to become greater. Shaw does not attack doctors as individuals in total control of their own fate. Indeed, he is among the pioneers of drama in taking them seriously: he sees them as victims of circumstance. He proposes to rescue them by shifting the emphasis to the promotion of health. A state medical service was to be controlled by a General Medical Council from which physicians would be excluded except as assessors and work under the jurisdiction of a Bureau of Statistics based on the ideas of Karl Pearson. One of Shaw's great criticisms of the medical profession was precisely its lack of attention to epidemiology (11, p. 27):

> It does happen exceptionally that a practising doctor makes a contribution to science (my play described a very notable one); but it happens much oftener that he draws disastrous conclusions from his clinical experience because he has no conception of scientific method, and believes, like any rustic, that the handling of evidence and statistics needs no expertness.

This lack of attention, like other deficiencies, arose from lack of time and lack of money.

Clearly it is only U.S. doctors who work in deprived areas and British junior hospital doctors who come near this description of the general practitioner of Shaw's day (11, p. 71):

> In other occupations night-work is specially recognized and provided for. The worker sleeps all day; has breakfast in the evening; his lunch or dinner at midnight; his dinner or supper before going to bed in the morning; and he changes to day-work if he cannot stand night-work. But a doctor is expected to work day and night. In practices which consist largely of workmen's clubs, and in which the patients are therefore taken on wholesale terms and very numerous, the unfortunate assistant, or the principal if he has no assistant, often does not undress, knowing that he will be called up before he has snatched an hour's sleep. To the strain of such inhuman conditions must be added the constant risk of infection. One wonders why the impatient doctors do not become savage and unmanageable, and the patient ones imbecile. Perhaps they do, to some extent. And the pay is wretched, and so uncertain that refusal to attend without payment in advance becomes often a necessary measure of self-defence, whilst the County Court has long ago put an end to the tradition that the doctor's fee is an honorarium. Even the most eminent physicians, as such biographies as those of Paget shew, are sometimes miserably, inhumanly poor until they are past their prime.

Again, Shaw comes near to anticipating the later criticism of the hospital in medical training when he writes (11, p. 22):

> A doctor's character can no more stand out against such conditions than the lungs of his patients can stand out against bad ventilation. The only way in which he can preserve his self-respect is by forgetting all he ever learnt of science, and clinging to such help as he can give without cost merely by being less ignorant and more accustomed to sick-beds than his patients. Finally, he acquires a certain skill at nursing cases under poverty-stricken domestic conditions, just as women who have been trained as domestic servants in some huge institution with lifts, vacuum cleaners, electric lighting, steam heating, and machinery that turns the kitchen into a laboratory and engine house combined, manage, when they are sent out into the world to drudge as general servants, to pick up their business in a new way, learning the slatternly habits and wretched makeshifts of homes where even bundles of kindling wood are luxuries to be anxiously economized.

However, I do not quote him here to praise his rightness in detail,[2] but to emphasize that he sees the problems of the organization of medical care within the context of society as a whole. This, paradoxically, is what the functionalist fails to do, as does his more sophisticated successor.

PARSONS—ACHIEVEMENTS AND LIMITATIONS

It must be remembered that the celebrated chapter 10 of Parsons' *The Social System* (14), part of which is so often quoted in discussions on the sick role, was an attempt precisely to relate medical activity to society as a whole. Furthermore, Parsons must be given full credit for two features of his analysis, namely his separation of motivation from structural factors, and his characterization of the sick role and the physician role in terms of similar pattern variables. Despite Parsons' clear awareness of complexities, and the complication of the language with which he tries to contain them, his basic theory tends to the simplification of reality rather than its classification. Thus in his essay "The Professions and Social Structure" (15), first published in 1939, he argues that both businessmen and professionals seek personal success, and that their differing actions (e.g. relatively unrestricted and relatively restricted advertising) reveal not the contrast of egoism and altruism as motivation, but their embeddedness in different structures of social action. They have in common achievement orientation, universalism, and functional specificity. They differ only, perhaps, in that the latter are collectivity oriented.

Parsons' starting point is to display that old wine which radical (what can be taken for granted) sociology is presently engaged in putting into old bottles, albeit with new labels. How does it come about, he asks, that physicians are able to require patients to obey them and to suffer privation, hardship, and even death on doctor's orders? Why is it taken for granted that patients should comply? First, because in our society like others there is a sick role, and second, because in our society unlike others there is a patient role. All societies have illness which either happens from outside or is created as a social state. "Illness may be treated as one mode of response to social pressures, among other things, as one way of evading social responsibilities. But it may also, as will appear, have some positive functional significance" (14, p. 431). An ill person moves into the sick role, which consists of "a set of institutionalized expectations and the corresponding sentiments and sanctions." Its characteristics are:

- A legitimated exemption from normal social role responsibilities. This exemption is a duty as well as a right.

- He is in a condition which needs to be remedied. He cannot help it but someone must help him.

- His state is undesirable and he and others should remove him from it as soon as possible.

- He is obliged to seek competent help to get himself out of it.

[2] Shaw himself says that his enthusiasm for Sir Almroth Wright and the opsonin theory may be overtaken by events (11, p. 84): "By the time this preface is in print the kaleidoscope may have had another shake; and opsonin may have gone the way of phlogiston at the hands of its own restless discoverer."

"It is [says Parsons] here, of course, that the role of the sick person as patient becomes articulated with that of the physician in a complementary role structure" (14, p. 437).

The Sacredness of the Physician

Now that Parsons has told us what is so special about the sick, he goes on to describe the physician, who (to Parsons) appears to be sacred in a Durkheimian sense. Parsons slides prematurely here into the assumption of identity between sick role and patient role, and defines the physician in terms of a unity of opposites—a sharing of values and pattern variables with the profane patient. The patient is controlled, ignorantly uncertain, the object of the death process. The physician controls, is wisely uncertain, is intimate with death. It is interesting, says Parsons (14, p. 445):

> ... to note that the dissection of a cadaver is included in the very first stage of formal medical training, and that it tends to be made both something of a solemn ritual, especially the first day, on the part of the medical school authorities, and medical students often have quite violent emotional reactions to the experience. It may hence be concluded that dissection is not only an instrumental means to the learning of anatomy, but is a symbolic act highly charged with affective significance. It is in a sense the initiatory rite of the physician-to-be into his intimate association with death and the dead.

The Boston women noticed this too in 1971 when they wrote (6, p. 239): "It is also interesting to speculate on the effect on doctors of their first contact with the human body in medical school—a corpse, the ultimate passive object."

Another feature of the physician's sacredness is his privileged access to secrets and secret places; the vagina and the rectum are specifically mentioned by Parsons as places where, in Parsons' world, even one's best friends are not admitted. (Compare again the Boston Women's injunctions (6) to explore oneself and others, and especially the photograph and text on p. 270.) For this and other reasons, physicians maintain their functional specificity. They scorn friendship and its diffuseness, they cling to their affective neutrality. Even the psychotherapist subject to transference puts it to cathartic not cathectic use.

The physician to fulfil his function seeks an Archimedean place to stand, a place from which to serve his patient without losing his role, or giving in to the patient's unconscious desire to have the physician as a love object, if only a father. (Parsons' explanation of the difference between stern fathers and kind psychotherapists is peculiarly revealing of the nonuniversality but class-period specificity of Parsons' whole analysis: "But when a son misbehaves a father reacts with anger and punishment, not affectively neutral "understanding" (14, p. 462).)

At this point, as he turns to a more detailed discussion of the last pattern element, collectivity-orientation, Parsons deals in passing with "certain theorists." Like patients who call cancer "that disease," Parsons rarely allows the words Marx or Marxists to pass his typewriter keys. Similarly, he always euphemizes the adjective capitalist to capitalistic. It is collectivity-orientation

> ... which is distinctive of professional roles within the upper reaches of our occupational system, especially in the contrast with business. Indeed one of the author's principal motivations in embarking on a study of the medical profession lay in the desire to understand a high-level occupational role which deviated from that of the businessman who, according to certain theorists, represented the one strategically crucial type of such role in modern "capitalistic" society (14, p. 463).

He then refers us to his essay, "The Professions and Social Structure" (15), which I have already mentioned and which to me, although not apparently to Parsons, shows precisely how similar physicians and businessmen are. As he himself later says in a rare purple passage (14, p. 473),

> It is a particularly vivid example of the importance of the sociological analysis of the social system for formulation of the problem of the analysis of motivation when the generalization of the implications of that analysis is to be extended beyond the single individual to problems of significance to the social system.

Parsons' Social Position and His Theoretical Deficiencies

In his theoretical conclusions, Parsons is at his most functionally optimistic and empirically wrong. He sees the latent functions of sick role, physician role, and their interaction as being concerned with social control and the "correction" of deviance. He distinguishes again between the patient role and the sick role, but fails to see all the implications of this. He writes (14, p. 477), perhaps correctly,

> The sick role is, as we have seen, in these terms a mechanism which in the first instance channels deviance so that the two most dangerous potentialities, namely, group formation and successful establishment of the claim to legitimacy, are avoided. The sick are tied up, not with other deviants to form a "sub-culture" of the sick, but each with a group of non-sick, his personal circle and, above all, physicians. The sick thus become a statistical status class and are deprived of the possibility of forming a solidary collectivity.

This may be true of the sick but it is not true of patients, nor has the sacredness of physicians lasted to the extent that the following statement (14, p. 445) carries any conviction today.

> It is interesting to note that even leftist propaganda against the evils of our capitalistic society, in which exploitation is a major keynote, tends to spare the physicians.

Parsons seems to me to be unable to separate himself from his own class position and hopes; unlike his ideal type physician, he fails to find an Archimedean place to stand. Such consistency as he manages to show, he achieves by leaving out of account the preventive and educational functions of medicine, by varying his level of comparison between professions, and by substituting piecemeal comparison for analytical history. Furthermore, he uses a concept of illness based, it would appear, on serious potentially mortal ailments. He shares the romantic view of physicians, and like many teaching hospital specialists, sees medicine in terms of peaks of either rarity or mortal crisis. Not for him Freidson's emphasis on the importance of the office atmosphere, nor the Boston Women's concern with daily tiredness or dysmenorrhea. Compare Mao's earthier approach (16):

> To allocate a great deal of manpower and resources to the study of difficult illnesses and to carry out penetrating research is to aim at the peaks to detach [medical work] from the masses. The result is to ignore or to assign only small amounts of manpower and resources to the prevention or care of common, frequent, widespread diseases. "Peaks" are not being abandoned, but they are going to receive less manpower and resources. The lion's share of manpower and equipment should be allocated to tackling the problems most urgently demanded by the masses.

Good advice to the sociologist as well as to the "Department of City Gentlemen's Public Health," as Mao suggested the ministry might be renamed.

Parsons and Sigerist on the Sick Role

The contrast between Parsons' analysis and Sigerist's careful historical siting of the special position of the sick is marked (5, pp. 9-22). These characteristics of Parsons' medical sociology are consistent with his ahistorical, contemporaneous orientation toward the American working class and their alleged permanent lack of militancy (14, p. 514). It is, however, important to note that Parsons is not always wrong, nor are his concepts useless. It is his sense of context—location in time and space—which is his weakness. He cannot see the classes for the roles—a position more dangerous than that of those mechanical Marxists who cannot see the roles for the classes, or that of the so-called radicals who see neither class, role, nor structure but only subjectively meaningful interaction.

FREIDSON'S VIEWS: MEDICAL SOCIOLOGY OR SOCIOLOGY OF MEDICINE?

Friedson, to whom I now turn in this regard, merely puts forward a pious hope (8, p. 3). Having referred, inter alia, to "the relation of the class system to the medical division of labor," he continues, "one may hope that sociologists, if not historians, may make more use of such material in the future."

Freidson, however, having stated the deficiencies of medical sociology so clearly, shows also most clearly the deficiencies of criticism. Following Straus, he makes a distinction between sociology in and of medicine. Sociology *in* medicine allows its problems uncritically to be defined not by sociology but by one status group within the profession, namely the doctors. "Medicine [he writes] may only be served, not evaluated" (8, p. 47). For this reason, the field is dominated by two kinds of study, social epidemiology and patient or prospective patient behavior. The subject is management oriented. This tendency is reinforced by the availability for study of patients and students and the concomitant nonavailability of high status "professionals." The possibility of escape from this frame of mind is hindered by both the medical ideology of professional skill *and* the sociologist's envy of it, which leads them to lean over backwards in their desire to be respectable. What is required, says Freidson, is a sociology *of* medicine; only then can the sociologist contribute meaningfully to social policy.

In Freidson's own words:

> In this book [*Professional Dominance: The Social Structure of Medical Care*] I shall examine medicine in general, but most particularly the medical profession and the institutions providing medical care from the point of view of the sociology *of* medicine. I shall attempt to show how, by adopting that point of view, one can better evaluate the nature of medical institutions in a way that is useful to the formulation of practical social policy. Indeed, I believe that only by adopting the perspective of a critical outside observer of medicine can one approach it in a way closely attuned to the public good, for *while medicine has a foundation in scientific knowledge, its characteristics as a social institution lead it inevitably to have a distorted view of itself, its knowledge, and its mission. Collaborating with medicine in its institutionalized tasks requires adopting that distorted view with all its deficiencies* [emphasis added]. Studying it as an outsider allows one to see medicine as one of a number of human institutions, reflecting merely one of many intellectual points of view, one of many moral standpoints, and expressing the material interests and ideological commitments of only one of many organized groups in our society. Once one sees medicine that way, one is in a good position to evaluate how far social policy should allow the profession to determine for itself the terms of the medical care it provides the public, and how far not (8, p. 42).

Like Shaw, Freidson's position leads him to see the organization of medical care as the central problem of medical sociology. It also leads him, perhaps, to substitute one set of gods (proper doctors, i.e. physicians) by another (clever doctors, i.e. sociologists). Alas, sociologists too exist within society. My italics, in the paragraph just quoted, could apply to sociology as well as to medicine. Let us, however, see where it leads Freidson.

Freidson is led by his initial dichotomy into a critical look at the structures of medical care and particularly at the part played by physicians as a *profession* in the process of social control within health services, as well as the social control exercised (or often not exercised) over physicians themselves.

The part of physicians in the delivery of medical care, he argues, makes it necessary for sociologists to see the profession not merely as an ethically based ideology into which individuals are socialized, "but as an occupation organized in a particular way, with stable relations to other occupations and standing in a particular relationship to its clientele. In essence, it must be seen as a status in society, participating in a division of labor and in given organizations. And the behavior of its members can be seen as a product of those structural relations" (8, p. 55). He is in fact surprisingly Parsonian!

The first contradiction Freidson sees within medicine is between its individualist ideology and reality. Sociology in medicine shares this ideology, and so sees the problem of medical care in terms of individual motives, whereas what is at issue is the social environment in which individuals work. No amount of good education and socialization will overcome the deterministic force of this environment. For example, he distinguishes, as Stein and Susser (17) also do, between client-dependent and colleague-dependent practice. The solo, fee-for-service practitioner in the U.S. has, he argues, to please his patients in order to survive, but is relatively independent of his colleagues.

The hospital doctor is under surveillance by his colleagues although controlled by a bureaucracy. However, in both cases the situation is in reality more complex. The pattern of practice and referral in the first case ensures the existence of an informal network of control by like-minded patients *and* colleagues of similar social class and ethnic background. This control has the effect of ensuring a uniformity of practice within a given social area, but not necessarily ensuring that it is good in any area. Within the hospital, matters become both more complicated and more theoretical. Freidson follows Parsons in pointing out that Weber's view of rational/legal authority was too simple. Weber neglected the fact that legitimate authority may be derived from expertise as well as or instead of from incumbency of office.

Freidson elaborates further to argue that, while the expertise of the scientist or nonmedical consultant depends on the persuasive powers of the individual expert over the individual client, in the case of the doctor it derives from his membership of the profession. This authority is related to class origin (8, p. 98), and is informally recognized and legally sanctioned in the United States and other industrial societies. The patient is encouraged neither to choose freely between licensed physicians and other healers, nor to answer back, nor even to understand what is happening to him. The physician is backed by law, custom, and indispensability. He is thought to have a monopoly of skill within the area. This entitles him to treat the patient as a non-person: as an object. This becomes most *apparent* in the long-stay mental hospital, as a large number of scholars, of whom Goffman is the most eloquent, have pointed out. It is actually at its sharpest and most acute, however, in the case of major surgery when the patient is deprived of human consciousness altogether. (Acupuncture "anesthesia" for this reason, I would argue, is systematically consistent with the amateurism of barefoot doctors: the patient remains subject not object.) Clients (and radicals) do not object and cry alienation to surgeons (although Shaw did the equivalent in the twenties) because they think surgery is effective. They do raise the cry against psychiatrists because they suspect that psychiatrists are treating people as objects to no good or even useful end.

The Virtues of Bureaucracy

The issue within the hospital centers on the contradiction between the bureaucratic administration and the professional autonomy of the physicians. In Freidson's view, bureaucracy should not here be an "epithet"; in a rational world bureaucracy needs strengthening against professionalism. The restriction of the freedom of the physician is the liberation of the patient (and incidentally of the nurse and the auxiliary). The therapeutic community in which patient, professional, pundit, parent, and administrator are equals in a community of healing is a utopian dream which is only dreamable in the mental hospital (and educational institutions) where the technology is soft, and it is unlikely to succeed even there. (In his survey of the literature, Freidson overlooks Rapoport's *Community as Doctor* (18) with its account of a partial success.)

Freidson Summarized

I can summarize Freidson's analysis in his own words in two paragraphs. The first (8, p. 155):

> In essence, my argument has been that the weaknesses to be found in professions are not mere flaws that can be corrected by recruiting better men, improving their training, and organizing their work more effectively. They cannot be eradicated by the profession itself. Those weaknesses are consequences of the fact that men cannot be led to serve an occupation by becoming committed to its ideals alone. They must also become committed to a concrete career and to concrete, historically located institutions. And in the case of professionals they also develop a sense of pride based on a typical conception of the special nature of their work. All three things, I suggest, compose professionalism, and in their interaction they produce the characteristic weaknesses of professions. *And since those weaknesses stem from professionalism itself, professions cannot be expected to be able to rectify them* [Freidson's emphasis].

Thus far, I can travel with Freidson, but he does not seem to me to go far enough. Why should professions have this weakness? Are there professions in precapitalist society, and need there be in postcapitalist society? And why does not a competent and critical sociologist like Freidson ask these questions? Sociology too is historically situated. Freidson's failure to ask these questions leads naturally to his practical conclusions (8, p. 160):

> In essence [once more], my position is that the delivery of medical care cannot be controlled by the profession, that its autonomy and its dominance must be tempered by administrative or bureaucratic mechanisms that stress accountability for effective and humane services and must be in some way more responsive to the lay client himself.

Freidson, unlike Parsons, perceives outside the limits of his social position; but like Parsons he cannot act outside it. He sees clearly the diminishing role of patient choice in both the hospital and ambulatory services. His solution is to transfer choice from profession to bureaucracy—while enabling the *individual* patient (not the organized patient) to influence events, through paying or withholding a fee-for-service. He hopes to restore choice by restoring competition. His radicalism is that of Disraeli rather than

Marx. He regrets the development of medicine parallel with the development of large-scale capitalism (19) and hankers for a return to modified laissez-faire, but with factory inspectors thrown in. A benevolent state must protect the public from monopoly.

He does not see whole but piecemeal, although the evidence is there in his own work that medical attitudes are consistent with the rest of society. Managers claim the expertise to manage, teachers to instruct, and the rich to rule. Each depends on the other.

Unlike the women of the Boston Health Collective (6, p. 242), Freidson does not put his reading of *Fortune* magazine (20) to good use:

> In the decade of the sixties the total dollars spent for all health care in the United States doubled, reaching the figure of $62 billion in 1969. It is expected that this will climb to $94 billion by 1975, and that the health industry will then be the nation's largest in dollar volume and number of people employed.

Freidson's attitude toward the mobilization of patients as a whole is most revealing. He writes (8, pp. 226-227):

> The . . . mobilization of patients themselves into organized action groups is, to my mind, a last resort, appropriate only when all other devices have failed and when services remain nonetheless rigidly unresponsive to patient needs. When patients are organized into such groups, issues become undesirably stereotyped and negotiation takes place in terms that are not likely to serve the mutual benefit of all parties. It would be a tragedy if medical (and, for that matter, educational and welfare) services were so deeply resistant to accommodation of client needs that confrontation politics became the rule of the day. I think it can be avoided by a properly designed system of care.

His criticism of society here deserts him. First of all he assumes there *is* a solution acceptable to *all* parties. Second, he fails to learn the lessons of the path trodden by sociologists of race relations, significantly now called black studies. Third, he shows a liberal fear of confrontation. Finally he assumes that a system of care can be designed independently of concrete group interests, falling into the same kind of fallacy as he rightly ridicules in those sociologists who see the solution to the problems of medicine simply in the reform of the medical school.

Freidson recognizes the problem of the individual but he does not see the essential paradox that there has to be a social answer to those individual problems. If both structuralist Freidson and functionalist Parsons fail to make this connection, the so-called radicals of the New Sociology are in an even less advantaged position to do so. The focus on individual interaction produces fascinating material and entertaining reading; Goffman (21) in the operating theatre and Emerson (22) on the lithotomy position are joys forever. But these observers do not in themselves take us nearer to an understanding of social relations which could guide our actions. After all, the gynecologist was behaving successfully in the same way before the micro-sociologist came into the theatre.

I am not arguing against such studies, nor against such pioneer work as that of Glaser and Strauss' *Awareness of Dying* (23). I am saying that for micro-sociology to be meaningful it must be put in a totalizing context.

MEDICAL SOCIOLOGY FOR WHOM?

It was Marx's custom when faced with a new phenomenon to ask himself the question, "cui bono?" or "to whom the good?" Who could then benefit or should benefit from a theory of sociology of medicine? To whom should we present the theory? The commonsense answer in the past has appeared to be to the doctors. We should present medical sociology in one form or the other in the medical school. This was the answer of

Jefferys (24) in 1969 and of Robinson (25) in 1973. There are two arguments in favor of such a strategy. If we can convince the doctors, they will use their prestige to convince the patients and we will be home and dry. Dry and well fed, since we can get paid at the same time. Freidson has shown us the academic danger of this position. Despite Parsons' injunction that we should not glibly assume (14, p. 467) that surgeons, for example, do unnecessary operations just for the money, as sociologists we must recognize the difficulty of getting people to act against what they perceive as their own interests.

Should we then seek an Archimedean point of leverage? Should we stand on the sidelines, above and beyond, and influence and control from there? But again we medical sociologists have nowhere independent to stand. We, too, have entrenched professional positions and a class origin and instincts to be reinforced. We share the elite tendencies of the physician, and we do not have even the skin contact with the mass of the population and the element of manual work that clinical practice brings. Success in sociology is manipulative, and sociologists past and present have sought manipulative solutions. Uncertain of success, like physicians, they have taken refuge like them in magic and mystification. If sociology is the opiate of the intellectuals, words are the opiate of the sociologists. When he described his concept of "total institutions" in *Asylums* (26), however, Goffman recognized an alternative: identification with the interest of the patients, as they see it, not as redefined in a medical mode. It is interesting that so much superior if not good social medicine should have emerged from South Africa, where it was relatively easy to disidentify with official policy (27). And interesting too that white South Africa could not tolerate it, and avoided its practitioners.

The clearest understanding of the realities of medicine in context came in the past from socialist vestryman Shaw of St. Pancras, and now from such bodies as the Boston Women's Health Book Collective. The confrontation which Freidson wishes to avoid is already latently there. McKinlay (28) reported in his study of "underusers" in Aberdeen that car travellers were regarded with suspicion. Only when he walked or cycled did he become acceptable. The car was perceived as a symbol of otherness by poor patients. The symbol could have been a white skin, a white coat, or a white mask.

> There is another curious thing. When a doctor examines a patient, he always covers his mouth with a gauze mask, whatever the patient's illness. Is he afraid of passing germs to his patient! I think he is more likely to be afraid of his patient passing germs to him. He must make a difference here [between the patients with infectious diseases and those without]. To wear a mask under all circumstances is to build a barrier between him and his patients.

So wrote Mao Tse-tung in his attack on the Ministry of Public Health in June 1965 (16).

Sociologic theory in the field of medicine as elsewhere must be alert to recognize conflicting interests and their symbols and to analyze the reasons for them in their context. This is the demystification function of science which must challenge professional autonomy. As Gill and Horobin (29) have pointed out, it may be that the resentment of and opposition to abortion by British doctors arises not so much out of piety and reverence for life as out of the threat to medical autonomy presented by patients who come to a doctor knowing what they want him to do, instead of asking for advice and direction.

Adopting a posture of alliance with patients is already a revolutionary step; it challenges the autonomy of the doctor. Pursued to its logical conclusion it is also, as implied in Sigerist's analysis, a challenge to the state. For the state is not interested in the health of its subjects (more properly, objects). Its interest lies in their not being sick; they can be ill but not sick. This is a quite different perspective from that of the patients themselves. Patients are anxious to get well again but prefer never to have been ill. People at large are more likely to believe that prevention is better than cure than are doctors, officials, or entrepreneurs. As the history of China shows, even a socialist ideology and economy has difficulty in putting a preventive medicine program consistently into practice. Even Freidson's administrators cannot manage such a program under capitalism against the authoritarianism of doctors, and the vested interests of drug companies, whether pharmaceutical, tobacco processing, or distilleries.

Furthermore, while Marx's descriptions of socially created disease, quoted above, seem remote and historical in the prosperous parts of western industrialized countries, in Southern Italy (30), Latin America, and elsewhere they still represent reality. Even in civilized England, with its National Health Service, class differentials in mortality seem to be widening (31) and availability of services is least where they are most needed (32). Medical sociologic theory needs to see these developments in historical context to avoid facile and ineffective suggestions for solution. Sociologists at least need to understand as Shaw did that physicians are, like capitalists and dominating parents, as much victims of the structures of which they form part as they are in some contexts to be seen as enemies. But what do they know of doctors that only doctors know? Health services seen in isolation may indeed suggest that physicians are the main barrier to improvement and change. The historical context may help us to avoid such dead-end theorizing as preferring fringe to scientific medicine and to avoid imagining, in a new humanistic form of Christian Science, that sickness has no reality but arises iatrogenetically like other forms of deviance through labelling. *Titulatus ergo sum* is then seen as an adequate defense against hospitalization as well as imprisonment.

In conclusion, let me reiterate that I do not wish to belittle the achievements, as far as they go, of empirical medical sociologists. It is medical sociology as integrative theory which is here under attack. The theory is too important to leave to Parsons or Freidson, or even sociology as a whole. Stacey (33) and Draper and Smart (34) can show their fellow sociologists and doctors that in the reorganized British National Health Service patients as a whole will have less power and influence. To be effective, they need to show politicians and patients as well, and to do this they need a theory. Oddly an art critic, who is also a Marxist, seems to me to state the problem more clearly than most (35, pp. 54-55).

> It is true that all works of art exercise an ideological influence—even works by artists who profess to have no interest outside art. . . . But having said that, one must differentiate between works which are intended to have an immediate and short-term effect and are expendable, and works which are intended to be more enduring.
>
> [Later he defines the difference:] The short-term works, which can justifiably be subsumed under propaganda, must reveal in their structure and form their urgent but temporary function. They should be like "orders of the day." If they are not, much of their necessary urgency is lost.
>
> Works which are intended to have a long-term effect need to be far more complex and to embrace contradictions which may allow them to survive. They need to be concentrated, not upon the isolated exigencies of the moment, which can only be made total by social action submitting to and mastering them, but upon the new, now imaginable totality which reality represents.

We should be grateful to Parsons and Freidson for seeking to make medical sociology realist rather than naturalist, art rather than propaganda. Alas, in sociology as in art, the illusion that you are neutral means you are on the wrong side.

REFERENCES

1. Foucault, M. *The Birth of the Clinic*. Pantheon, New York, 1973.
2. Marx, K. *Capital*, Vol. 1, edited by F. Engels. Allen & Unwin, London, 1946.
3. Lenin, V. *The Development of Capitalism in Russia*, Ch. 4, p. 254. Collected works, 3, English Ed. Foreign Languages Publishing House, Moscow, 1972.
4. Sigerist, H. *Socialised Medicine in the Soviet Union*, Ch. I, pp. 24-80. Gollancz, London, 1937.
5. Roemer, M. I., editor. *Henry E. Sigerist on the Sociology of Medicine*, pp. 9-22, 65-74. MD Publications, Inc., New York, 1960.
6. Boston Women's Health Book Collective. *Our Bodies, Ourselves*. Simon and Schuster, New York, 1973.
7. Wootton, B. The law, the doctor and the deviant. *Br. Med. J.* 2: 197-202, July 27, 1963.
8. Freidson, E. *Professional Dominance: The Social Structure of Medical Care*. Atherton Press, Inc., New York, 1970.
9. Zola, I. K. Medicine as an institution of social control. *Sociol. Rev.* 20(4): 497-504, 1972.
10. Boxill, R. *Shaw and the Doctors*. Basic Books, New York, 1969.
11. Shaw, G. B. *The Doctor's Dilemma*. Penguin Books, Harmondsworth, 1946.
12. Shaw, G. B. *Everybody's Political What's What*, Ch. 24, pp. 213-225. Constable, London, 1944.
13. Shaw, G. B. *Doctors' Delusions*. Constable, London, 1932.
14. Parsons, T. Social structure and dynamic process: The case of modern medical practice. In *The Social System*, Ch. 10, pp. 428-479. Routledge & Kegan Paul, London, 1951; The Free Press, Glencoe, Ill., 1951.
15. Parsons, T. The professions and social structure. In *Essays in Sociological Theory*, rev. ed., Ch. 2, pp. 34-49. Free Press, New York, 1954.
16. Ch'en, J. *Mao Papers: Anthology and Bibliography*, p. 100. Oxford University Press, London, 1970.
17. Stein, Z., and Susser, M. Hypothesis: Failures in medical care as a function of the doctor's situation. *Med. Care* 2(3): 162-165, 1964.
18. Rapoport, R. N. *Community as Doctor. New Perspectives on a Therapeutic Community*. Tavistock Publications, London, 1960; Charles C Thomas, Springfield, Ill., 1960.
19. Stern, B. J. *Historical Sociology*, pp. 395-400. Citadel, New York, 1959.
20. Myers, H. B. The medical industrial complex. *Fortune* 90-95, January 1970.
21. Goffman, E. *The Presentation of Self in Everyday Life*. Penguin Books, Harmondsworth, 1971.
22. Emerson, J. Behavior in private places: Sustaining definitions of reality in gynecological examinations. In *Recent Sociology No. 2: Patterns of Communicative Behavior*, edited by H. P. Dreitzel. Macmillan, New York, 1970.
23. Glaser, B. G., and Strauss, A. L. *Awareness of Dying*. Weidenfeld & Nicolson, London, 1966.
24. Jefferys, M. Sociology and medicine: Separation or symbiosis. *Lancet* 1: 1111-1116, 1969.
25. Robinson, D. *Patients, Practitioners and Medical Care*. Heinemann Medical Books, London, 1973.
26. Goffman, E. *Asylums. Essays on the Social Situation of Mental Patients and Other Inmates*. Anchor Books, Garden City, New York, 1961; Penguin Books, Harmondsworth, 1968.
27. Kark, S. L., and Steuart, G. W. *A Practice of Social Medicine*. Livingstone, Edinburgh and London, 1962.
28. McKinlay, J. B. Some Aspects of Lower Working Class Utilization Behavior. Unpublished Ph.D. dissertation, Aberdeen University, 1970.
29. Gill, D. G., and Horobin, G. W. Doctors, patients and the state: Relationships and decision making. *Sociol. Rev.* 20(4): 505-520, 1972.
30. Macciochi, M. A. *Letters from within the Italian Communist Party to Louis Althusser*. New Left Books, London, 1973.
31. Preston, B. The statistics of inequality. *Sociol. Rev.* 22(1): 103-118, 1974.
32. Tudor Hart, J. The inverse care law. *Lancet* 1: 405-412, 1971.
33. Stacey, M. Consumer Complaints Procedure in the National Health Service. Unpublished paper to British Sociological Association, Medical Sociology Group, York, 1973.
34. Draper, P., and Smart, T. *The Future of Our Health Care*. Report on the current proposals for the re-organisation of the National Health Service. Guy's Hospital Medical School, London, 1972.
35. Berger, J. *Art and Revolution*. Penguin Books, 1969.

CHAPTER 3

The Industrialization of Fetishism or the Fetishism of Industrialization

A Critique of Ivan Illich

Vicente Navarro

According to the media and other organs of popularization, our Western developed societies are in crisis. Thus, the number of analysts and synthesizers providing remedies to this crisis is proliferating. One of them is Ivan Illich, Director of the Centre for Intercultural Documentation in Cuernavaca, Mexico. Widely quoted and debated, he has been variously defined as the genius who provides the focus for our doubts (1), a revolutionary who gives the best prescription for change (2), and a "petit réactionaire" who is nostalgically looking for Bucolia (3). But whatever characterization may best apply to Illich, he is an articulate theoretician and one of the more recent in a long roster of builders of what I consider to be the most prevalent and influential ideology used to explain our societies, i.e. the ideology of industrialism. As such, his work merits serious response.

Assuming that the best way to understand an author's analysis of our reality is by first comprehending the ideological framework on which that analysis is based, let me begin by summarizing very briefly the main characteristics of the ideology of industrialism of which Illich's writings are part and parcel. I will then describe how those characteristics appear both in his analysis of our Western developed societies and of our health services as well as in his normative synthesis, i.e. the basis for his strategy for change. In both cases the main, but not only, point of reference will be Illich's most recent book, *Medical Nemesis* (4).[1] In the second part of this chapter I will discuss the assumptions underlying Illich's ideology and will analyze the degree to which they provide valid explanations of

---

[1] This book has been briefly summarized in the *Lancet* (5) and in *Social Policy* (6). Unless otherwise indicated, the references to Illich's *Medical Nemesis* are to the book (4) and not to its summaries.

the actual situation in our Western developed countries and in our health services. Where the explanations are found to be invalid, I will present alternate explanations of the social problematique of our countries. And in the third part, in light of those alternative explanations, I will discuss the extent to which Illich's recommendations for change are relevant to the solution of our problems.

INDUSTRIALISM AS IDEOLOGY AND ITS PRESENTATION IN ILLICH'S WRITINGS

Industrialism is the most prevalent ideology used to explain the nature and form of our Western developed societies. Grounded largely in technological determinism it owes much to Max Weber, and it suggests that the industrial nature of technology defines social organizations in their entirety (7).

Among the primary characteristics of that ideology is that the production requirements of the technological process and, pari passu of industrial organizations, are the most important determinants of the nature and form of our Western developed societies, i.e. industrialized societies. In a fatalistic and almost deterministic way the former—the technological process—leads inevitably to the latter—the industrialization of society. Moreover, according to the theorists of industrialism, that industrialization has transcended and made irrelevant and passé the categories of property, ownership, and social class. Indeed, ownership loses its meaning as legitimization of power. And control, now assumed to be divorced from ownership, has passed from the owners of capital—the capitalists—to the managers of that capital, and from there to the technocrats, those who have the skills and knowledge needed to operate the major social edifices of industrialism, the bureaucracies. The new elite, then, are the bureaucrats, who have supplanted the capitalists. Within this evolution, a new social order based on bureaucracy has transcended the capitalist order. Capitalist societies have thus become industrial, postindustrial, and mixed-economies societies. As Frankenberg (8) has indicated, words such as capitalism, social class, and related ones rarely pass through these theoreticians' typewriter keys, except in an introductory note of dismissal.

Also, according to the theoreticians of this ideology, in this evolutionary process of industrialization, there is a disintegration of the old preindustrial order, assumed to be integrated, self-sufficient, and communal. In the words of Illich (4, p. 65), because of industrial growth "social arrangements allowing such autonomy [of community members] have practically disappeared." And in the industrial order that replaces it only the values that are functional for the "formal rationality" of the system are sustained and replicated; productivity, efficiency, progress, and modernization are the components of the intellectual-philosophical construct of the ideological building of industrialism. Basic requirements of that construct are the need for hierarchy and dependency within those hierarchies. At the top of that hierarchy is the expert, the bureaucrat; at the bottom is the subject of that bureaucracy, the receiver or consumer of the goods, commodities, or services administered by that bureaucracy. Within this hierarchy the former manipulates the latter, in theory for the benefit of both, in practice for the benefit of the former more than the latter.

A final characteristic of industrialism is that it claims to be a universal process. In other words, all societies, regardless of their political structure, will evolve according to the dictates of industrialization. Indeed, according to a key component of that ideology, *the theory of convergence,* all societies will progress toward the urban-industrial model of the future. Thus, socialism and capitalism are usually seen as two convergent roads to the same destination, "the industrial model." In the words of one of its most successful popularizers (9),

> Such reflection on the future would also emphasize the convergent tendencies of industrial societies, however different their *popular or ideological billing,* the convergence being to a roughly similar design for organization and planning. . . . Convergence begins with modern large-scale production, with heavy requirements of capital, sophisticated technology, and, as a prime consequence, elaborate organization [emphasis added].

The ideologists of industrialism then, including Illich, predict the inevitable development of societies of a unitary type, leading to an urban-industrialized model. In that respect, the history of the human race is the history of the different stages of development toward that model. Accordingly, the degree of development of any country is measured by the extent to which it approximates that model, with the United States being held as the most developed country, i.e. closest to that model.[2]

Viewed in this way, the social problems of society (the U.S.) become not the problems of capitalism (an altogether passé category), but the problems of industrialization. And I tend to suspect that the great prevalence of that ideology throughout our society, including academia, can be explained partially by its self-flattering interpretation of our problems, i.e. the social problems we face result from our pioneering the great search for modernization, and from being ahead in our industrialization. Ours, in summary, is the burden of the leaders. In the words of an influential popularizer in the U.S., "We have to pay the social investment of being the first. Others will learn from our failures and successes" (13).

If one accepts this ideology, it then makes sense to study and analyze the social problematique of the already industrialized societies, primarily of the U.S., to see how much other less-developed countries can learn from both their successes and failings. Ivan Illich, director of one academic center physically situated in a developing country, Mexico, focuses the attention of all his writings on the industrialized societies, with greatest emphasis on the U.S. Consequently, he draws most of his references from and bases most of his categories on Western developed countries.

If there is general agreement among the theoreticians of industrialism, at least on the main assumptions summarized above, there is far less agreement on the conclusions they draw. Indeed, while some like Daniel Bell (14) and Walt Rostow (10) rejoice over the fruits of industrialization, others like Raymond Aron (15) seem to have second thoughts, and others still, such as Illich (16), despair and try to rebel. Unless we reverse industrialization, writes Illich (5, p. 921), ours will be a "compulsory survival in a planned and engineered Hell." Not surprisingly, then, their suggestions for change differ widely. But an approach increasingly heard, and one that Illich seems to share, can be defined as that of Jeffersonian republicanism which recommends (a) the debureaucratization of our

---

[2]The most representative theoretician of this stage theory is Rostow (10). For a critique of Rostow's stages with special emphasis on their implications in the health sector, see reference 11. Another work that presents this model is that of Kahn and Wiener (12), in which the level of development of the countries is measured by the estimated number of years that it will take for those countries to reach the 1965 U.S. level of overall economic development, measured by the ubiquitous gross national product per capita.

society; (b) the reversal of industrialization and growth with the breaking down of professional and other monopolies toward a return to the free market of goods and services; and (c) a renewed emphasis on the self-reliance and autonomy of the individual, with enlightened self-interest as the prime mover in his relationships of exchange.

Industrialism in Illich's Writings

The ideology of industrialism, placing the credit and in Illich's case the blame for our social development and its problematique on the inevitable process of industrialization, underlies the theoretical constructs used by most analysts of our Western society, including its critics, such as Illich.

Indeed, Illich believes that industrialism is the main force shaping our societies and that unavoidable "rising irreparable damage accompanies industrial expansion in all sections" (5, p. 920), including medicine (4), education (17), and so on. For example, the industrialization of medicine leads to the creation of a corps of engineers—the medical profession—comparable to the technocrats of the main social formation of industrialized societies, the bureaucracy. Thus, the industrialization of medicine means its professionalization and bureaucratization. Moreover, and reflecting the assumed universality claimed by the ideology of industrialism, Illich believes that all societies, either capitalist or socialist, converge toward the same model, following a similar evolutionary process. Indeed, "the frustrations [due to industrialization] which have become manifest from private-enterprise systems and from socialized care have come to resemble each other frighteningly" (5, p. 921). The same problematique that appears in Houston is likely to appear in Moscow, in Bogotá to appear in Havana, and in Taiwan to appear in People's China as well. The differences in the expression of that problematique are more quantitative, depending on the level of industrialization and stage of development of those countries, than qualitative. Capitalism and socialism are indeed outmoded concepts, since they are basically converging toward the same path of industrialization that overwhelms and directs their social formations.

In this interpretation, then, the class conflict has been replaced by the conflict between those at the top, the managers of the bureaucracies, indispensable to the running of an industrialized society, and those at the bottom, the consumers of the products—goods and services—administered by those bureaucracies. As applied specifically to medicine, that conflict is the one between the medical bureaucracy, primarily the medical profession and the medical care system, and the consumers, the patients. This antagonistic conflict appears as iatrogenesis (damage done by the provider), and it is

> clinical, when pain, sickness, and death result from the provision of medical care; it is social, when health policies reinforce an industrial organization which generates dependency and ill health; and it is structural, when medically sponsored behaviour and delusions restrict the vital autonomy of people by undermining their competence in growing up, caring for each other and aging (4, p. 165).

The first and most documented type of iatrogenesis is the clinical one, damage done by the physicians and providers of services, and is caused primarily by their engineering approach to medicine in which the individual is seen as a machine, an aggregate of different pieces that have to be put right through therapeutic intervention. Adding to that cause, there is also much injury that is due simply to much arrogance, sheer incompetence, and misunderstanding of what health is about (4, pp. 15-25).

Social iatrogenesis is the addictive dependency of the populace on the medical care institutions. Indeed,

> public [demand and] support for a nationwide addiction to therapeutic relationships is pathogenic on a much deeper level, but this is usually not recognized. More health damages are caused by the belief of people that they cannot cope with illness without modern medicines than by doctors who foist their ministrations on patients (4, p. 39).

In that respect,

> the proliferation of medical institutions, no matter how safe and well engineered, unleashes a social pathogenic process. Over-medicalization changes adaptive ability into passive medical consumer discipline (4, p. 39).

According to Illich, the cause for that addiction is the manipulative behavior of the medical bureaucracy that perpetuates and encourages that passive and addictive consumer behavior. In this scheme of things the power of that bureaucracy is its exclusive and monopolistic power of definition of what is health and what method of care may be publicly funded.

Last but certainly not least, *structural iatrogenesis* is the loss of autonomy of the patient and the creation of his dependency. In this iatrogenesis, the medical bureaucracy goes further than creating addiction, and destroys "the potential of people to deal with their human weakness, vulnerability and uniqueness in a personal and autonomous way" (4, pp. 87-150). According to Illich, the responsibility for health and care is taken away—expropriated—from the individual by the medical industry. Moreover, this structural iatrogenesis is assumed to be intrinsic in the values and modus operandi of the medical industry and civilization. Thus the intervention of the medical industry has the same effect as that of any other industry, i.e. it breaks with those social values and cultures, such as acceptance of death, disease, and pain, assumed to be in existence in the preindustrial societies and that are capable of providing the self-realization of the individual (4, p. 160).

Illich's Strategies for Change: The Debureaucratization and Deindustrialization of Society and Medicine

How can we avoid and correct these iatrogeneses, the extensive damage done by the industrialization of medicine? Before stating his own solutions, Illich briefly considers several other alternatives presently debated in the political scene. In discussing solutions for *clinical* and *social iatrogeneses,* he especially rejects the "socialization alternative" that he attributes to the "equalizing rhetoric" of the misleadingly called progressive forces, among which he includes liberals and Marxists. According to his normative conclusion, the redistribution of medical care implied in the socialization alternative would make matters even worse since it would tend to further medicalize our population and create further dependencies on medical care (4, p. 66). Indeed, "less access to the present health system would, contrary to political rhetoric, benefit the poor" (4, p. 73). In that respect, Illich finds the creation of the National Health Service in Britain as a regressive, not progressive, step.

Instead of socialization and its implied redistribution, Illich recommends the following solutions for clinical and social iatrogeneses:

- The mode of production in medicine should be changed via its deprofessionalization and debureaucratization to break down the barriers that allow the "disbursement of any such public funds under the prescription and control of guild members" (4, p. 121). In that respect he suggests what Friedman (18) and Kessel (19, 20) have proposed in this country, that licensing and regulation of healers should disappear, and the concerns of where, when, how, and from whom to receive care should be left to the choice of the individual.

- Collective responsibility for that care should be reduced and individual responsibility should be maximized. Self-discipline, self-interest, and self-care should be the guiding principles for the individual in maintaining his health. In summary each one should be made responsible for his own health. Indeed, Illich's dictum in health sounds very close to the dictum of another theoretician of the virtue of self-reliance, Ex-President Nixon's "don't ask what the state can do for you, but what can you do for yourself" (21).

As to structural iatrogenesis, the most important of the three, and the one that Illich especially attributes to industrialism, he again dismisses the alternative of the socialization and public control of the process of industrialization, recommending instead the reversal of that process, i.e. breaking down the centralization of industry and returning to the market model. According to Illich, "only the inversion of society's overall growth rate in marketed goods and services can permit a reversal" (4, p. 160). And within this competitive market model, the motivations for social interaction will be those of enlightened self-interest and a desire for survival (4, p. 164). The essence of his strategy for correcting structural iatrogenesis, then, is an anti-trust approach with strong doses not of Marx, or even Keynes, but of Friedman.

A CRITIQUE OF ILLICH AND AN EXPLORATION OF ALTERNATIVES

Clinical Iatrogenesis: The Illusion of Doctors' Effectiveness

Perhaps not surprisingly, most of the debate on Illich's writings on medicine has focused on his postulate that individual clinical intervention may be doing more harm than good (clinical iatrogenesis). Actually, not only medical journals such as *The Lancet* in Britain, but popular magazines like *Le Nouvel Observateur* in France have focused primarily on Illich's skepticism about the therapeutic value of medical intervention. In this skepticism he follows the by now well established and known tradition of non-medical writers such as Montesquieu, Tolstoy, Bernard Shaw, and many others who had questioned the effectiveness of the professionals' tasks throughout the passing of decades. Unfortunately, the medical profession has dismissed too frequently and too uncritically those questions as being too perverse and frivolous to merit serious consideration. And the inquiring minds within the profession that kept asking the same questions and providing evidence to support such skepticisms were and still are equally dismissed or boycotted as unwelcome prophets of an unwelcome change. (For a further discussion of this point see reference 22.)

Illich, in a short but meaningful review of what he defines as the effectiveness of medical care, summarizes the available information on the effectiveness of some therapeutic interventions, and thus provides evidence on the limitations of those interventions. Not unexpectedly, he is more pessimistic about the value of those interventions than most clinicians would be, but paradoxically is far more optimistic about the effectiveness of some of those interventions, e.g. for skin cancer treatment or early surgical intervention for cervical cancer (4, pp. 16-19), than most health care researchers would be (see, for example, Holland (23)).

Still, he adds his iconoclastic voice (a welcome voice, I might add) to an increasing chorus of doubters of the effectiveness of medical tasks. A major weakness of his evaluation, however, is that he takes as an indicator of the effectiveness of medical *care*, indicators of *cure*. Indeed, he seems to confuse care with cure. And in evaluating the effectiveness of medical care he does what most clinicians—Illich's engineers in the medical system—do; he analyzes the degree to which medical intervention has reduced mortality and morbidity, i.e. the effectiveness of health care intervention in *curing* disease and avoiding mortality. But, at a time when the most important type of morbidity in our Western developed societies is chronic, a much better indicator of the effectiveness of the medical *care* intervention would be the way that care is provided in that intervention, i.e. the degree to which the system provides supportive and attentive care to those in need. And the limited evidence available does seem to indicate that medical *care* may make a difference, i.e. it may reduce disability and discomfort in people's lives. (For a sketchy review of this *care* effectiveness, see reference 24.) But for that taking *care* to occur, our medical care system would have to change very profoundly to better enable the system to provide that care.

Still, since Illich seems to see an inevitable progress toward the present cure-oriented system, he does not seem to accept or even welcome the possibility of creating another system in which the priorities would be opposite to those of the present ones, with emphasis given to care as opposed to cure services. Actually, Illich would not welcome such a care-oriented system since it would increase the dependency of the individual on the physician and on the system of medical care, preventing the much-needed self-reliance and autonomy. Indeed, according to Illich, whatever good medical cure or care may do is certainly outbalanced by the damage that it creates. And he finds the greatest damage to be the dependency that medical care creates in the population, i.e. social iatrogenesis.

Social Iatrogenesis: Addiction to Medical Care Institutions, Cause or Symptom?

Illich considers social iatrogenesis, the addictive behavior of the population to medical care, to be the result of manipulation by the medical bureaucracy—the medical care system. It is a manipulation that aims at creating dependency and consumption. Indeed, Illich postulates that the consumer behavior of our citizenry is primarily determined by its manipulation by the bureaucracies created as a result of industrialization. Allow me to focus on this postulate, and to discuss the consumer behavior of our citizenry, not only in the health sector of our economy but in all others as well. Disagreeing with Illich, I find that manipulation of addiction and consumption by bureaucracies (including the medical care bureaucracy) is not the cause, as he postulates, but the symptom of the basic needs of the economic and social institutions of what he calls industrialized societies, but what I would call industrialized capitalist societies.[3] Actually, I consider those bureaucracies, be

[3] In this chapter capitalist societies are societies in which, notwithstanding the existence of a "public sector," the largest majority of economic activity is still dominated by private ownership and enterprise that primarily benefits a dominant class. In those societies, the state owns only a subsidiary part of the means of production. As Miliband (25) writes, to speak of "mixed economies" in those societies is to attribute a special and quite misleading meaning to the notion of mixture.

they trade, services, or "whatever," to be the mere socialization instruments of those needs, i.e. they reinforce and capitalize on what is *already* there—*the need for consumption,* consumption that reflects a dependency of the individual on something that can be bought, either a pill, a drug, a prescription, a car, or the "prepackaged moon." Indeed, the overall quantum of citizens' dependency is far more than the mere aggregate of dependencies of those citizens on the bureaucracies of our societies. Actually, those dependencies are mere symptoms of a more profound dependency that has been created in our citizenry not by industrialization, but by the capitalist mode of production and consumption—a mode of production that results in the majority of men and women in our societies having no control over the product of their work, and a mode of consumption in which the citizenry is directed and manipulated in their consumption of the products of that work. (For excellent reports on how the values are being shaped in our societies, see references 26-28.) As Marcuse (29) had indicated, that system makes people aspire to more when this more must always be inaccessible. This dependency on consumption—this commodity fetishism—is intrinsically necessary for the survival of a system that is based on commodity production. It is then necessary for the owners and controllers of the means of production of that system to stimulate dissatisfaction and dependency in the sphere of consumption. Thus, those owners and controllers must provoke continual artificial dissatisfactions and dependencies in human beings that direct them toward further consumption because without them the system would collapse. And, as I will try to show later, Illich's bureaucracies, including the medical bureaucracies, are not the generators, but the administrators of those dependencies, consumptions, and dissatisfactions. Indeed, those bureaucracies are not the owners nor the controllers, but the administrators of that system.

In summary, in this alternate explanation, addiction and dependency on consumption—either of goods or services—is not due primarily to the manipulative behavior of bureaucracies, but is the result of the basic needs of an economic system that requires for its survival (a) the creation of wants, however artificial or absurd they may be, (b) the existence of a passive and "massified" population of consumers, and (c) the replication of consumer ideology whereby the citizen is judged not by what he *does* (his work) but by what he *has* (his consumption). Within that system, the citizen, the consumer, is made to believe that his fulfillment depends in large degree on his consumption, be it of drugs, pills, prescriptions, cosmetics, and whatever may be required for his fitness, well-being, and pursuit of happiness. Within this scheme of things, to consider that need for consumption, that addictive behavior, to be the result of bureaucratic manipulation is (a) to underestimate the needs of the economic system, and (b) to far overestimate the role of those bureaucracies. Theirs is, again, the task of administering and reinforcing that dependency on consumption that is *already there*.

Let me underline here that I do not deny the powerful effect that Illich's bureaucracies, such as the medical and related bureaucracies, e.g. drug advertizing, have on administering and reinforcing (but not creating) a harmful demand for their goods and services. But I don't believe that the disappearance of those bureaucracies (if it were at all possible) from our capitalist societies would mean the disappearance of that addictive demand. Indeed, Illich's focus on the world of consumption and his theories of manipulation ignore the main determinants of people's behavior, which are not in the sphere of consumption, but in the world of production.[4] Indeed, in our capitalist system

---

[4] Also, Illich's focus on the addictive part of medical care consumption seems to ignore a valid need for medical care responsive to the needs for both cure and care of our population.

what the individual might have (defined in the area of consumption) depends on what he might do (defined in the world of production). Indeed, whatever he can buy depends very much on how much money he makes. And for the great majority of our citizens, the amount of money they make depends primarily on what type of work they do and how much they are paid for it. Thus, to understand the *sphere of consumption* we have to understand the *world of production,* or who does what, who controls that work, and how that control takes place. And an analysis of that world of production shows the following: (a) The great majority of producers—the workers—do not have much control over the nature and product of their work. What they do in the workplace and how they do it is, in the great majority of cases, outside the control of the workers, and within the control of the employer. (b) Work is for the majority of producers primarily not a means of self-expression, where creativity is the goal, but a means to get income to be able to buy the services and goods necessary to satisfy their needs. The most important components in one's life, creativity and worthiness, are not realized in one's daily work. In other words, the worker must spend time at work to get freedom and capacity for development outside the sphere of production and work. Ironically, this hope for fulfillment during leisure time turns out to be an illusion, an illusion that has to be satisfied with the always unsatisfied and never-ending consumption. In summary, denied of his self-realization at his place of work, the world of production, the worker then has to look for that realization in the sphere of consumption. The alienation of the producer from his work—his dissatisfaction—leads to the fetishism of consumption. (For an elaboration of the concept of alienation, see references 30 and 31.)

Actually, the whole concept of worker alienation had been discussed in the sixties as irrelevant to the actual conditions and perceptions of the working class. Moreover, the ubiquitous Gallup Polls showing that the majority of workers were satisfied with their work seemed to confirm that perception. As Wright and others have shown, however, those results represented more the biases of the researchers than the views of the interviewees. When the questions were phrased differently it appeared that the feelings of helplessness, withdrawal, alienation, malaise, and pessimism were not minority but majority sentiments among substantial sections of the working class, primarily among the young workers, to such a degree as to become an industrial problem (see the Senate testimony of James Wright, Director, National Policy Affairs, National Center for Urban Ethnic Affairs, quoted in 32, pp. 29-35). As Walter Dance, Vice President of General Electric, indicated

> We see a potential problem of vast significance to all industrial companies. . . . This involves the slowly rising feeling of frustration, irritation and alienation of the blue collar workers; the "hard hats," if you will, but not just the activists in big cities (quoted in 33, p. ii).

Subsequent studies such as the report on *Worker Alienation, 1972* of the Committee on Labor and Public Welfare of the 92nd United States Congress (32) show that alienation is prevalent, among not only blue, but also white collar workers. And, as the report of a special task force to the U.S. Secretary of Health, Education, and Welfare, entitled *Work in America* (34) indicates, a main reason for those producers' alienation is the limiting effect of the nature of their work and their powerlessness to change it.

The response to that situation—the limiting effect of work—varies depending on the degree of awareness and consciousness of the individual to that situation. And, one increasingly important response is the expression of that dissatisfaction in labor conflicts. Actually, the number of working days lost in the U.S. due to labor strikes concerning issues of working conditions—the nature of work—exceeds those concerning the size of the paycheck or the amount of fringe benefits (35). For an excellent account of the alienation of the working class, the majority of the U.S. population, see "The Discontent of Work," in Levison (36).

Another reaction to that alienation is, as Dreitzel (37) has pointed out, its internalization, appearing as a major cause of psychosomatic illness, the type of problem most frequently presented to the medical care system. Indeed,

> doctors from various industrialized countries unanimously report that at least 50 per cent of their patients suffer from "functional disturbances," i.e. illness without any establishable organic cause (37, p. viii).

Thus, in the medical care system we also find that (a) the alienation of the individual in his world of production leads him to the sphere of consumption, the consumption of health services, and that (b) the medical care bureaucracy is just administering those disturbances created by the nature of work and the alienating nature of our system of production. Actually, the increasing awareness of this phenomenon explains the choice by the American Public Health Association of "Work and Health in the U.S." as the main theme for its 1975 Annual Meeting. As an editorial of the journal of that Association (38) indicates, work is the keynote, not only of the restoration of health but also of the maintenance of health in our society. Actually, that editorial repeats what Albert Camus wrote somewhat more elegantly, "Without work all life goes rotten. But when work is soulless, life stifles and dies" (quoted in 34, p. xx).

In summary, Illich's focus on consumption leads him to believe that the loss of autonomy (including the expropriation of his health) and subsequent dependency of the individual are due to the manipulation and effect of the bureaucracies in the individual's sphere of consumption. Disagreeing with him, I believe that the loss of autonomy and the creation of dependency start in the producer's loss of control over the nature, conditions, and product of his work—the expropriation of his work. Indeed, according to my postulate, the loss of autonomy of the citizen does not start in the sphere of consumption but in the world of production.

Bureaucratization of Work: A Product of Industrialization or of Class Control?

Another consequence of focusing on the world of consumption and not on the area of production and its class relations is that it leads Illich to misunderstand the nature of bureaucracy and bureaucratization of work in our societies. He just assumes that technological knowledge and the all-pervasive industrialization determine a division of labor that explains the appearance of production, trade, and services bureaucracies. But this explanation begs the questions of why that technological knowledge is distributed in the way that it is, and why that technology is frequently a vehicle of human oppression and not of liberation. Indeed, I would postulate that technology is not an independent force that fatalistically determines all relations, including social ones, but rather the reverse is true, i.e. the social relations (who controls what, and how this control takes place) determine the type of organization to be chosen and the type of technology to be used. As Braverman (39) has shown, (1) a historical review of "what preceded what" shows that the managerial revolution—Taylorism—and the bureaucratic form of organization that it created preceded the scientific revolution and not vice versa; and (2) that bureaucratic form of organization was and is created by the need of the employer—the manager—to structure and control the process of work. Indeed, that control is a major power of the employer. And characteristics of that structure and control are that (1) decision making has to be organized from the highest levels downwards, according to a vertical order of hierarchy in which the only ones who have complete control and a "complete picture" of the process of production are the controllers of that process; (2) technologies employed must (a) enable, be compatible with, and replicate that hierarchical division of labor, and (b) fragment the nature of work, making every producer an expert of a small part—but not the whole—of the process; and (3) the distribution of technologies, skills, and knowledge must, within the constraints of (1) and (2), be compatible with the minimization of costs and the maximization of profits (40).

Within that process of production, technology and its requirements do not determine the hierarchical division of labor, but the hierarchical division of labor determines the type of technology used in that process. Technology, then, reinforces the already existing hierarchical and fragmentary division of labor. Indeed, that hierarchicalization is already there and is determined primarily by the class and sex roles existent in our societies. Let me illustrate this with an analysis of the responsibility that the members of the health team have. Within that health team, we find a well-defined hierarchical order with the physician, most often a man of upper-middle-class extraction, at the top; below him, the supportive nurses, most often women with lower-middle-class backgrounds, and at the bottom, under both of them, we find the attendants and auxiliaries, the service workers, who most frequently are women of working-class backgrounds.[5] According to Illich and other industrialist theorists, what primarily explains that hierarchy are the different degrees of control over the technological knowledge necessary for the provision of industrialized medicine. But past and present experience shows that (a) the responsibilities that the different members of the team have are primarily due to their class backgrounds and sex roles, and only secondarily, very secondarily indeed, to their technological knowledge;[6] and (b) this technological knowledge, far from causing that cleavage and hierarchy among these members, merely reinforces that hierarchy. In that respect the acquisition of that knowledge—education and training—is the mere legitimation of that class and sex hierarchical distribution of power and responsibilities (41). Indeed, although the degree of technological knowledge developed in medicine has changed dramatically since the Flexner Report of 1910 to the present, the class composition of the members of the health team has not changed significantly from that time[7]. Actually, the Flexnerian "revolution" in medicine and the creation of scientific medicine further strengthened but did not create that class distribution of responsibilities within the health sector that already existed. Indeed, to assume, as Illich does, that the distribution of responsibilities in medicine is due to its industrialization is to confuse symptoms with causes. It is *primarily* the class structure and the class relations

---

[5] In this categorization, working class includes blue collar, service, and farm workers. For a class analysis of the labor force in the health sector, see reference 41.

[6] Actually, due to the rapid rate of obsolescence of the technological knowledge in medicine, it is not infrequent to find knowledge to be more dysfunctional than functional.

[7] Let me clarify in this footnote that I do believe there have been profound changes in the structure and composition of the labor force, including the labor force in the health sector. But most of these changes have taken place within each social class, not among social classes. For a further elaboration of this point, see reference 41.

of our society that determine that distribution. And, one could further postulate that this class structure and hierarchy militate against the provision of comprehensive medical care. For example, while most of the needs of the patients in our populations are those of care, most of the strategies within the health team and the health sector are directed by the "expert" in cure, the physician. The strategy for care within that team, however, would require (a) not the authoritarian (vertical), but the collaborative (horizontal) distribution of responsibilities, and (b) not a change from experts in cure to experts in care, but rather giving the team—including *all* its members as well as the patient—responsibility for both care and cure. However, the joint provision of the care, by the patient himself, his family, and all members of the team, is seriously handicapped in our class-structured society, where roles and functions are not distributed according to the need for them, but primarily according to the hierarchical order prevalent in our society, dictated by its class structure and class relations.

Structural Iatrogenesis: Industrialism or Capitalism?

Illich, by dismissing from the very beginning the categories of capitalism, class structure, and class relations, is seriously limited in finding the causes of his structural iatrogenesis. Indeed, while he attributes clinical iatrogenesis to the physicians, and social iatrogenesis to the medical care system, he finds structural iatrogenesis to be due to the culture of industrialization. Structural iatrogenesis, Illich writes, "is spawned by a cancerous delusion about life, and manifests itself when this delusion has pervaded a culture" (4, p. 160). And the creation of that culture that pervades "medical industry and civilization" is the symptom of the overall and pervasive process of industrialization. His solution for that iatrogenesis includes (a) reversing industrialization and its growth rate, (b) breaking down industrial bureaucracies, starting with the medical one, and (c) returning to self-reliance and enlightened self-interest. And in this struggle against industrialization and bureaucratization it is of paramount importance to start with medicine,

> since medicine is a sacred cow, its slaughter would have a "vibration effect": people who can face suffering and death without need for magicians and mystagogues are free to rebel against other forms of expropriation now practiced by teachers, engineers, lawyers, priests and party officials (4, p. 161).

But, by focusing on the medical bureaucracy as the "enemy," Illich misses the point because those bureaucracies are the servant of a higher category of power that I would define as the dominant class. Indeed, the empirical analysis of the health industry shows that contrary to what Illich believes, that industry is administered but not controlled by the medical profession. The analysis of power in the health sector in most Western developed societies shows that that power is primarily one of class not of professional control. Indeed, those who have the first and final voice in the most important "corridors of power" in the health sector are the same corporate groups (composed mainly of the upper, corporate, or capitalist class) that control and/or have dominant influence in the organs—Illich's bureaucracies—of production, consumption, and legitimation in our societies. Indeed, as I have shown elsewhere,[8] members of the corporate class (owners and managers of financial capital), the class that has a dominant influence in the most

---

[8]For a detailed presentation of the available evidence on the social class composition of the decision-making bodies in the U.S. health sector, see reference 41.

important spheres of the U.S. economy—the monopolistic sector—have a dominant influence as well in the funding and reproductive institutions of the health industry (commercial insurance agencies, foundations, and teaching institutions). And members of the upper-middle class (executive and corporate representatives of middle-size enterprises and professionals, primarily corporate lawyers and financiers) have dominant influence in the delivery institutions. A similar situation appears with the executive and legislative branches of federal government that oversee and regulate the activities in the health sector. And in all these top agencies of power, the medical profession is represented only to a small degree. Indeed, the medical bureaucracy administers but does not control the health sector. And its power is delegated to it from the corporate and the upper-middle classes. Those classes and the medical profession share similar but not identical corporate and class interests, and if a conflict appears—and, as I postulate elsewhere (41), such conflict is bound to appear—then, it is quite clear who has dominant control in that situation, the same ones who have had that control from the *very beginning*, the corporate or dominant class. Indeed, one has to remember that the supporters and sponsors of "Flexnerian scientific medicine" were the Rockefeller and Carnegie Foundations, the voices of the corporate class of that period.

We find then that the main conflict in the health sector replicates the conflict in the overall social system. And that conflict is primarily not between the providers and consumers, but between those that have a dominant influence in the health system (the corporate class and upper-middle class) who represent less than 20 per cent of our population and control most of the health institutions, and the majority of our population (lower-middle class and working class) who represent 80 per cent of our population and who have no control whatsoever over either the production or the consumption of those health services (41). To focus then, as Illich and the majority of social critics do, on the conflict between consumers and medical providers as the most important conflict in the health sector, is to focus on a very limited and small part of the actual class conflict.

Actually, Illich's dismissal of the concept of social class as an irrelevant category for his analysis leads him to see the conflict in a compartmentalized way, i.e. as taking place among individual holders of skills and trades on the one hand, and the supposed benefactors of those skills and trades, the consumers, on the other. Thus he sees the "campagne dé bataille" in the control and redefinition of those skills and trades. But here again the conflict seen in this way begs the questions of (a) why those skills and roles are distributed in the way they are to begin with; and (b) why those skills and roles are very frequently vehicles more of oppression than liberation.

Regarding the first, the distribution of skills and roles in the medical sector, Illich assumes that what gives power to the medical profession is the exclusive control of those skills and trades, thus his suggestion of deprofessionalization. My answer however, is, as I have indicated, that those skills and trades reinforce and legitimate the power that is *already* there. The deprofessionalization of medicine and the dehierarchicalization of medicine, i.e. its democratization, are not possible within our class-structured society. The change of the latter is a prerequisite for the change of the former. The reverse, as Illich suggests, is unhistorical.

As to the frequently oppressive role of the medical bureaucracies, Illich considers that they fail and determine oppression because they generate a self-serving addiction. His unawareness of social class structures and relations as the most important conceptual framework for understanding our institutional behavior, including the medical institutions, prevents him from understanding that services bureaucracies—including medicine—are, far from failing, succeeding in what they are supposed to do. Indeed, had Illich's analysis been historical and dialectical, he would have understood that the functions of the health industry are primarily determined outside and not inside the health sector. As Susser (42) has written, the concepts of health and of the types of health services have continuously changed and been redefined according to the needs of the capitalist mode and relations of production. And in this process of redefinition, the ones that have the dominant voice in defining health and health services have not been the medical bureaucracies as Illich writes, but the dominant class—the capitalist or corporate class. For example, when the economic needs (productivity of the system) and political needs (quieting social unrest) of that class so required in Britain, that class supported and passed the national health insurance of Lloyd George's government in 1911 in spite of the opposition of the medical profession (42). And today, as then, most of the changes in the definition of health and health services have occurred not because but in spite of the medical profession. A recent example has been the change of therapeutic practice in obstetrics with the provision of abortion on demand. That redefinition of health practice was due to the needs of the organs of legitimation—including the juridical organs—to respond to (a) an increasingly alienated and radicalized women's liberation movement, and (b) the population policies of the time.

In all these cases the redefinition of values, or what Galbraith (43) calls the convenient social virtues, followed the needs of the corporate class, not of the medical profession. Indeed, as Galbraith has recently indicated, the convenient social virtues are the ones that are primarily convenient to the most powerful in our society. Actually, what Galbraith and others are increasingly saying was said quite clearly by Marx (44):

> The ideas of the ruling class are in every *epoch* the ruling ideas: i.e. the class which is the ruling *material* force of society, is at the same time its ruling *intellectual* force. The class which has the means of material production at its disposal, has control at the same time over the means of mental production.

And health values and ideas are not an exception.

According to this explanation, then, the medical profession is a repository and guardian of the definition of those values, but not the ultimate definer. Reflecting the actual location of power, the profession has continuously lost its battle against that redefinition whenever its power had to be tested in a conflict with the corporate and dominant class.

In summary, and as I have shown elsewhere (41), one of the functions of the services bureaucracies—including the medical bureaucracy—is to legitimize and protect the system and its power relations. One aspect of that protection is social control—the channeling of dissatisfaction—which Illich introduces as structural iatrogenesis. But, to believe that social control is due to the culture of medicine and the pervasiveness of industrialization is to ignore the basic question of who controls and most benefits from that control. An analysis of our societies shows that the services bureaucracies—including the medical ones—although willing accomplices in that control, are not the major benefactors. The ultimate benefactor of any social control intervention in any system is the dominant class in that system.

*A Final Note on the Convergence Theory: The Possible
Replication of Class Relations in Socialist Societies*

As I have indicated, the main feature of the theory of convergence is that all societies, either capitalist or socialist, are converging toward similar social formations, i.e. industrialized societies. And these societies are held to be characterized by a similar process of industrialization that has determined the predominance of the bureaucracy as the primary social formation, with managers and technocrats having replaced the dominant classes in those societies. The supporters of that theory give the USSR and the Eastern European countries as examples of socialist societies which because of their high degree of industrial development also have full-fledged bureaucracies as the controllers of social and economic activity in each sector, and thus increasingly resemble our own Western industrialized societies.

This analysis, however, is too much of a simplification. Indeed, an analysis of the Eastern European societies, including the USSR, shows that the bureaucracies—including the medical bureaucracies—are not the primary controllers of each social and economic activity, but are subservient to a larger authority, the political party. Indeed, the planning, regulatory, and administrative responsibilities of the state bureaucracies are subject to the higher power of the upper echelons of the party. And these higher echelons of the party are the ones that have created the state bureaucracies, not vice versa. The power of the party is manifested and expressed through those bureaucracies. In this alternate explanation of bureaucratization of Eastern European societies, that bureaucratization was not the result of industrialization, but the result of the party's need to control the process of production and industrialization. And that party became a dominant class in itself when (a) it began to use its control over the means of production, not to optimize the producers' control over the process and means of production, but rather to optimize the production itself, i.e. when the accumulation of capital became the primary goal of those societies; and (b) it used its political control over the production, trade, and services bureaucracies not to decentralize and democratize them but to optimize its control by increasing the centralization and hierarchicalization of those bureaucracies.

As Sweezy has indicated, it was the belief of the political party in the 1920s, shared by both Stalinists and Trotskyites, that (a) democratization of the process of production was impossible in an underdeveloped society, and that (b) the need for capital accumulation had to be the first priority in the thirties and forties in preparing for and winning the Second World War. It was primarily these beliefs that led to the centralization of power that created bureaucratization and absence of institutional democratization. (For an extensive elaboration on this point, see the debate between Sweezy and Bettelheim presented in reference 45; see also Sweezy (46).) As Sweezy and Bettelheim have indicated, the appearance of a dominant class—the party, and its servants—the bureaucracies, determined the replication of class relations between dominant and dominated classes which were similar to, although not identical with, those in Western societies. In this process, the state bureaucracies were and are the administrative agencies of those relations, but did not generate those relations. Indeed, as Bettelheim (45, p. 46) says "there cannot exist a 'state power of the bureaucracy,' because a bureaucracy is always in the service of a dominant class."

In summary, in those Eastern European societies the bureaucracy is subject to and dependent on the political power of the party. And although there is considerable overlapping of membership among both, still, the bureaucrat and technocrat are both formally and informally dependent on the dominant class, the political party. The democratization of the former would require the democratization of the latter. Indeed, the struggle for institutional and industrial control that took place during the Cultural Revolution in China (which included a battle against elitism and bureaucratization in the medical sector) was part of a far wider and more important conflict, i.e. the conflict between large segments of the peasantry and the industrial working class and a sector of the political party that had ceased to be representative and had become instead an oppressive dominant force, a dominant class (47). Similarly in Cuba, the fight against bureaucratization in the middle sixties that Che Guevara stimulated was one component of a wider political conflict against a sector of the leadership of the Communist party—the Escalante group—that wanted to give priority to capital accumulation and to the efficiency of the system, over the democratization of the system (48).

And, in still another example, in Chile, the conflict in the health sector between large segments of the population and the majority of Chilean medical professionals, led by the Chilean Medical Association, was part of a far larger conflict over the socialization and democratization of the society. And the opposition of the medical profession to Allende was not because Allende reduced the amount of technology available to it, as Illich seems to believe, but because, in encouraging the democratization of the health institutions, he was a threat to the perpetuation of its social class as well as professional privileges. Indeed, when Illich (4, pp. 42-43) writes that

> by far the majority of Chilean doctors resisted the call of their President [to reduce the national pharmacopoeia]; many of the minority who tried to translate his ideas into practical programmes were murdered within one week after the take-over by the junta on September 11, 1973,

one has to realize that the savage assassination of the physicians and other health workers who supported Allende by the military junta (with the assistance of the majority of the Chilean medical profession), was an action far transcending the irritation over a reduction of technology. Illich's primary focus on technology, to the degree of making a fetish of it, seems to make him unaware of the fact that the fight in Chile was one, not primarily over technology, but over the class control of the health and all other institutions. Indeed, as I have indicated elsewhere (49), the majority of the medical profession in Chile reacted as much, if not more, against the curtailment of their class as of their professional privileges.

Actually, the experience in the socialist societies does not show, in my opinion, that capitalism and socialism converge, but that (a) the socialization of the means of production is a necessary but not sufficient condition for its democratization; (b) the class structure and class relations may reappear and be perpetuated in socialist societies, not because of industrialization, but because of the political centralization of power; (c) the conflict and struggle against bureaucratization and for democratic institutional control that occurred in China, Cuba, and Chile were part of a far larger and more important one, i.e. the struggle for the disappearance of class structures and for the political and economic democratization of those societies; and (d) to the degree that class control of the health institutions changed, the product and nature of those institutions changed. Indeed, even the definition and meaning of health changed from one where health was seen as an individual effort motivated by enlightened self-interest, to one of community and collective effort.

FINAL COMMENTS ON THE POLITICAL RELEVANCE OF ILLICH

The Industrialization of Fetishism or the Fetishism of Industrialization

Having made a critique and review of Illich's writings, with primary focus on the area of health, and having postulated alternatives to both his explanations and his solutions, allow me to finish with some random thoughts about the political nature and relevancy of his two main suggestions for change: the reversal of industrialization, and the importance of self-reliance. In other words, a final note on the political uses and misuses of Illich's main messages.

As to the reversal of industrialization, I find Illich's emphasis on the process of industrialization as the culprit of his pains (iatrogeneses) quite a limiting one. Actually, by considering the industrialization and bureaucratization of our societies as the cause and not the symptom of our distribution of economic and political power, Illich seems to reduce all our political problems to managerial ones. In this way, he who resents the industrialization of all fetishism—including medicine—ends by fetishizing the process of industrialization itself. This fetishizing of that process appears, for example, in his analysis of the most important public health problem in the world today: undernutrition. Here, once again, Illich assumes that industrialization is the major cause of the problem.

> Beyond a certain level of capital investment in the growing and processing of food, malnutrition must become pervasive ... [and] what is happening in the sub-Saharan Sahel is only a dress rehearsal for the encroaching world famine. This is but the application of a general law. When more than a certain proportion of value is produced by the industrial mode, subsistence activities are paralysed, equity declines and the total satisfaction in that particular area diminishes. In other words, beyond a certain level of industrial hubris, Nemesis *must* set in (4, pp. 155-156).

Absent in this analysis is the consideration of the critical political factors of who controls those economies (land and capital) and the process of industrialization. By focusing on the process of industrialization per se, and avoiding the economic and political conditions that determine underdevelopment and the type of industrialization that is used (the inter- and intra-country conditions of economic exploitation, the control of international trade, and other factors), his analysis seems aseptic and almost neutral. But, an alternative explanation to that of Illich's for underdevelopment and malnutrition is that certain types of industrialization (e.g. the Green Revolution) ostensibly exported from capitalist countries have reinforced and capitalized upon, but not generated, the already existing maldistribution of economic and political power, both within and among nations, the actual causes of their underdevelopment. Actually, Cuba and China, two of the very few countries in the sphere of underdevelopment that have controlled and almost solved their malnutrition problem, had to break with that maldistribution of power to allow them to use industrialization differently, not for the benefit of the few, but for the benefit of the many. The real problem the progressive forces in those countries faced in solving their malnutrition problem was not the process of centralized industrialization, but the centralization of economic and political power in the dominant oligarchies, allied with the corporate transnational interests, which determined that centralized industrialization. To change the latter they had to break with the former. Actually, the priest Camilo Torres in Colombia, who was assassinated while trying to change those economic and political structures, understood the causes of underdevelopment and malnutrition in Latin America far better than the urbane, sophisticated Ivan Illich in Mexico.

Indeed, the experiences in both China and Cuba would seem to indicate that the type of industrialization that exists in developing countries is a symptom but not a cause of their problems. (For an elaboration of this point, see reference 11.) In spite of these realities, endless interpretations of the political phenomena of underdevelopment are being advanced and sold, either under the pretense of the "population problem," or more recently, of the "problem of industrialization," that do not clarify but further obfuscate the actual economic and political causes of underdevelopment, whose reality and existence are increasingly clear for all to see.

The Limitations of Doing One's Own Thing

We are left then with Illich's second major suggestion for solving our problems: the self-reliance, self-care, independence, and autonomy of the individual citizen. But what is the meaning of this self-care? This aspect of Illich's strategy for change appears to me to be close, if not identical, to the strategy of that segment of American youth that joined in the "Woodstock nation," a strategy that basically relies on "life-style" solutions. And in that strategy, "doing one's own thing," or in Abbie Hoffman's words, "whatever the fuck we want" (quoted in 50), is not only the goal, but also the means for change, i.e. freedom and liberty defined as the lack of social constraints.

I postulate that the popularity of this strategy in our U.S. social environment and its appeal to the organs of legitimation—primarily the media—is because, rather than weakening, it strengthens the basic ethical tenets of bourgeoisie individualism, the ethical construct of capitalism where one has to be free to do whatever one wants, free to buy and sell, to accumulate wealth or to live in poverty, to work or not, to be healthy or to be sick. Far from being a threat to the power structure, this life-style politics complements and is easily co-optable by the controllers of the system, and it leaves the economic and political structures of our society unchanged. Moreover, the life-style approach to politics serves to channel out of existence any conflicting tendencies against those structures that may arise in our society.

Similarly, we find this life-style politics appearing increasingly in the health sector. Self-care and changes in life style are supposed to be the most important strategies to improve the health of our individual citizens. And behavioralists, psychologists, and "mood" analyzers are put to work to change the individual's behavior. In the words of one advocate of this approach,

> It is becoming increasingly evident that many health problems are related to individual behavior. In the absence of dramatic breakthroughs in medical science the greatest potential for improving health is through changes in what people do and do not do to and for themselves (51).

This strategy of self-care, however, assumes that the basic cause of his sickness or unhealth is the individual citizen himself, and not the system, and therefore the solution has to be primarily his and not the structural change of the economic and social system and its health sector. Not surprisingly, this emphasis on the behavior of the individual, not of the economic system, is welcomed and even exploited by those forces that benefit from the lack of change within the system. Interestingly, here in the health sector we again find the same analysis and strategies for change that we found in the sixties in the analysis of poverty in America. The sociological studies, for the most part, focused their analysis on the poor, not on the economic system that produced poverty. Thus, not paradoxically, most of the strategy for eradicating that poverty—the anti-poverty programs—was directed at the poor themselves, but not at the economic system that produced that poverty. Let me clarify that, today, we have even more poor people than we had before those programs started and the effect of those programs has been very limited indeed.

Similarly, in the health sector, a plethora of behavioral and sociological studies are devoted to analyzing the behavior of the individual, but very few studies exist that concern the behavior of the economic and political system that determines that behavior to start with. And most of the strategies for change are focused on changing the behavior of the individual and not the behavior of the system; thus, the appearance of self-care and health education strategies as possible and plausible strategies for change. But a far better strategy than self-care and changes in life style to improve the health of the individual, would be to change the economic and social structure that, according to my postulate, conditioned and determined that unhealthy individual behavior to start with. Let me give a specific example: the problem of the unhealthy diet of our citizens. The strategy of the life-style politics for correcting the unhealthy diet of our population, by individually changing the food consumption patterns (diet) of individual persons, avoids the political question of why the individuals consume that diet in the way they do. Thus, it ignores the enormous power of the economic needs of specific corporate interests in (a) determining that consumption, and (b) stimulating a certain type of production. Indeed, as Dr. Meyer (52), Professor of Nutrition from Harvard, has indicated, a primary responsibility for the very poor diet of the U.S. citizens are the corporate practices of the food conglomerates (for a presentation of the relationship between corporate practices of these main food corporations and the diet of children, see reference 53). And these food conglomerates, as several studies have shown, are increasingly linked with the main sources of financial capital in this country, the most important sector of the corporate class and the one that has a dominant influence in most of the sectors of our economic system, a system, incidentally, that determines a set of priorities in which $2.5 billion dollars are annually being spent on pet food (54), while "26 million Americans cannot afford to purchase an adequate diet; and over 11.2 million of them receive no help whatever from any federal food program" (55).

In the light of this iatrogenic economic and political environment, and the overwhelming power and influence of those economic groups, to speak of changes in life style as the proper strategy sounds to me to be not only very limited and unrealistic, but naive and sheer escapism. Indeed, I would postulate that unless the patterns of ownership and control of the means of production and consumption of the food and all other industries and sectors change in our society, from the control by the few to the control by the many, we will continue to have as poor a diet as we have today and have had in the past. And, thus, contrary to what Illich and others postulate, I believe that the greatest potential for improving the health of our citizens is not primarily through changes in the behavior of individuals, but primarily through changes in the patterns of control, structures, and behavior of our economic and political system. The latter could lead to the former. But the reverse is not possible.

Actually, it is precisely because of the impossibility of the reverse, and thus the lack of conflict between Illich's message and the basic tenets of our economic system, that his message, the life-style politics, is and increasingly will be presented by the organs of the media as the resolution of our crises and problems.

Indeed, Illich, radical in style but intrinsically conservative in message and substance, will be paraded as part of our solution. And at a time of increasing crises in our societies, the change in life styles, as opposed to political change, will be paraded as the solution. Indeed, I predict that powerful organs of value generation will be extremely sympathetic to Illich's emphasis on cultural as opposed to political change, stirring "new hopes in the hollow breast of at least one jaded revolutionary" (56). Cultural revolution will indeed be used to further postpone political change. And meanwhile, I postulate that to the same degree that the cultural politics of the Woodstock nation proved easily co-optable and irrelevant to the solutions of our problems in the sixties, this cultural revolution in our society will be similarly co-optable and equally irrelevant to the problems of our nation in the seventies. History will tell.

Acknowledgments—I want to express my deepest appreciation to Janet Archer, Christopher George, and Linda Heath for assisting in the preparation of the manuscript.

REFERENCES

1. Cohen, N. M., and Backett, E. M. Medical nemesis. Book Review of *Medical Nemesis* by I. Illich. *Lancet* II(7895): 1503-1504, 1974.
2. Kozol, J. Quoted in I. Illich, *Deschooling Society*. Calder and Boyars, London, 1971.
3. Schwarzenberg, L. Le "bon sens" de Monsieur Illich. *Le Nouvel Observateur* 523: 3, 1974.
4. Illich, I. *Medical Nemesis: The Expropriation of Health*. Calder and Boyars, London, 1975.
5. Illich, I. Medical nemesis. *Lancet* I(7863): 918-921, 1974.
6. Illich, I. Medical nemesis: The destructive force of professional health care. *Social Policy* 5(2): 3-9, 1974.
7. Blackburn, R. A brief guide to bourgeois ideology. In *Student Power*, edited by A. Cockburn and R. Blackburn, pp. 163-213. Penguin Books, Baltimore, 1969.
8. Frankenberg, R. Functionalism and after? Theory and developments in social science applied to the health field. *Int. J. Health Serv.* 4(3): 411-427, 1974.
9. Galbraith, J. K. *The New Industrial State*, p. 389. Houghton-Mifflin, Boston, 1967.
10. Rostow, W. W. *The Stages of Economic Growth*. Cambridge University Press, Cambridge, 1962.
11. Navarro, V. The underdevelopment of health or the health of underdevelopment. *Int. J. Health Serv.* 4(1): 5-27, 1974.
12. Kahn, H., and Wiener, A. J. *The Year 2,000*. Macmillan, New York, 1967.
13. Cronkite, W. Report on industrialization. CBS News, August 1973.
14. Bell, D. The post-industrial society: A speculative view. In *Scientific Progress and Human Values*, edited by E. Hutchings and E. Hutchings. American Elsevier, New York, 1967.
15. Aron, R. *Progress and Disillusion: The Dialectics of Modern Society*. Praeger, New York, 1968.
16. Illich, I. *Tools for Conviviality*. Calder and Boyars, London, 1971.
17. Illich, I. *Deschooling Society*. Calder and Boyars, London, 1971.
18. Friedman, M. *Capitalism and Freedom*. University of Chicago Press, Chicago, 1962.
19. Kessel, R. A. The A.M.A. and the supply of physicians. *Law and Contemporary Problems* 35: 267-283, 1970.
20. Kessel, R. A. Price discrimination in medicine. *Journal of Law and Economics* 1: 20-53, 1958.
21. Nixon, R. M. U.S. Presidential Address, 1972.
22. Navarro, V. From public health to health of the public: The redefinition of our task. *Am. J. Public Health* 64(6): 538-542, 1974.
23. Holland, W. W. Taking stock. *Lancet* II(7895): 1494-1497, 1974.
24. Haggerty, R.J. The boundaries of health care. *Pharos* 35(3): 106-111, 1972.
25. Miliband, R. *The State in Capitalist Society: An Analysis of the Western System of Power*, p. 10. Weidenfeld and Nicolson, London, 1969.
26. Schiller, H.I. *Mass Communications and American Empire*. Beacon, Boston, 1971.
27. Schiller, H.I. *The Mind Managers*. Beacon, Boston, 1974.
28. Servan Schreiber, J. L. *The Power to Inform*. McGraw-Hill, New York, 1974.
29. Marcuse, H. *One Dimensional Man*. Beacon, Boston, 1964.
30. Ollman, B. *Alienation*. Cambridge University Press, London, 1974.
31. Pappenheim, F. *The Alienation of Modern Man*. Monthly Review Press, New York, 1974.

32. *Worker Alienation, 1972.* Hearings before the Subcommittee on Employment, Manpower, and Poverty of the Committee on Labor and Public Welfare, United States Senate, 92nd Congress. U.S. Government Printing Office, Washington, D.C., 1972.
33. Sheppard, H. L., and Herrick, N. Q. *Where Have All the Robots Gone? Worker Dissatisfaction in the '70's.* The Free Press, New York, 1972.
34. Special Task Force to the Secretary of Health, Education, and Welfare. *Work in America.* M.I.T. Press, Cambridge, Mass., 1973.
35. Zernan, J. Organized labor versus "the revolt against work": The critical contest. *Telos* 21: 194-206, 1974.
36. Levison, A. *The Working Class Majority.* Coward, McCann, and Geoghegan, New York, 1974.
37. Dreitzel, H. P., editor. *The Social Organization of Health.* Macmillan, New York, 1971.
38. Howe, H. F. Health and work. Editorial. *Am. J. Public Health* 65(1): 82, 1975.
39. Braverman, H. *Labor and Monopoly Capital: The Degradation of Work in the Twentieth Century.* Monthly Review Press, New York and London, 1974.
40. Marglin, S.A. What do bosses do? The origins and functions of hierarchy in capitalist production. *The Review of Radical Political Economics* 6(2): 60-112, 1974.
41. Navarro, V. Social policy issues: An explanation of the composition, nature and functions of the present health sector of the United States. *Bulletin of the New York Academy of Medicine* 51(1) second series: 199-234, 1975.
42. Susser, M. Ethical components in the definition of health. *Int. J. Health Serv.* 4(3): 539-548, 1974.
43. Galbraith, J. K. *Economics and the Public Purpose,* p. 31. Houghton-Mifflin, Boston, 1972.
44. Marx, K. The German ideology. In *Selected Works,* Vol. 1, p. 47. Lawrence and Wishart, London, 1962. (Quoted in C.H. Anderson, *The Political Economy of Social Class,* p. 60. Prentice-Hall, Englewood Cliffs, N.J., 1974.)
45. Sweezy, P., and Bettelheim, C. *On The Transition to Socialism.* Monthly Review Press, New York and London, 1971.
46. Sweezy, P. The nature of Soviet society. *Monthly Review* 26(6): 1-16, 1974.
47. Bettelheim, C. *Cultural Revolution and Industrial Organization in China: Changes in Management and the Division of Labor.* Monthly Review Press, New York and London, 1974.
48. Boorstein, E. *The Economic Transformation of Cuba.* Monthly Review Press, New York and London, 1968.
49. Navarro, V. What does Chile mean: An analysis of events in the health sector before, during and after Allende's administration. *Health and Society, Milbank Mem. Fund Q.* 52(2): 93-130, 1974.
50. Silber, I. *The Cultural Revolution,* p. 58. Times Change Press, New York, 1970.
51. Fuchs, V. Health care and the United States economic system. *Milbank Mem. Fund Q.* 50(2, part 1): 211-237, 1972.
52. Meyer, J. Interview, FM-WMG Washington Radio Station, September 1974.
53. Cornely, P. B. The hidden enemies of health and the American Public Health Association. *Am. J. Public Health* 61(1): 7-18, 1971.
54. The great American animal farm. *Time,* pp. 58-64, December 23, 1974.
55. Citizens' Board of Inquiry into Hunger and Malnutrition in the United States. *Hunger U.S.A. Revisited,* p. 9. National Council on Hunger and Malnutrition and the Southern Regional Council, Atlanta, 1973.
56. Toynbee, P. Quoted among press opinions of Illich's works, I. Illich, *Medical Nemesis,* p. 184. Calder and Boyars, London, 1975.

PART 2

The Political Economy of Health Care

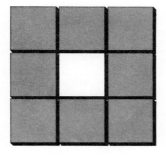

CHAPTER 4

Health Care in
the United States:
Who Pays?

Thomas S. Bodenheimer

The single most striking fact about the American economy is the vast disparity between rich and poor. The richest 20 per cent of the population receives 41 per cent of the total national income whereas the poorest 20 per cent receives 5.6 per cent (1). This inequality has not changed since 1910. In fact, the income gap between the average income of the poorest and the richest 20 per cent of the population was $10,500 in 1949, and $19,000 in 1969. The distribution of wealth (income plus assets such as real estate, stocks, bonds, and savings) is even more favorable for the rich. The top 20 per cent of the population owns over 75 per cent of the country's wealth, the wealthiest 8 per cent owns 60 per cent, and the super-rich 1 per cent owns 26 per cent. Twenty-five per cent of the population, on the other hand, owns nothing—their debts are at least equal to their assets.

Governments have an enormous influence on the distribution of income and wealth. This power is exercised through the collection of taxes and through the spending of public money. If taxes are collected principally from the rich and if government programs benefit the poor, wealth is thereby redistributed toward greater equality. If, on the other hand, taxes place a heavy burden on the poor and working classes, and if public funds are paid as subsidies to the rich, then the unequal distribution of wealth is perpetuated or worsened.

In 20th century America, governments have clearly perpetuated the radically lopsided distribution of income and wealth and thus have contributed to the maintenance of poverty. The mechanisms used by the government to maintain poverty are (a) excessive collection of taxes from poor and working-class people and sparing of

This chapter is an adaptation of Chapter 4 of *Billions for Bandaids. An Analysis of the U. S. Health Care System and of Proposals for Its Reform*, edited by Elizabeth Harding, Tom Bodenheimer, and Steve Cummings. Copies of this work, published by the Medical Committee for Human Rights in 1972, may be obtained from the Committee, P.O. Box 7677, San Francisco, California, 94119 at a cost of $2.25. Other topics discussed in the book include national health insurance, Health Maintenance Organizations, and the drug and insurance industries.

the rich from taxation, and (b) payment of significant amounts of public money as subsidies to large corporations, thereby benefiting the rich.

These matters are of critical importance to health care for two reasons. First, national health insurance—by taxing working people and bringing profits to rich providers and financers of care—will constitute another arena in which money is transferred from poorer to richer people. Second, the poverty which is inherent in maldistributed wealth is a major cause of death and disability in the United States.

WHO PAYS FOR HEALTH SERVICES?

At present, health care costs hit lower income people harder than richer people. In 1963, the average family earning $2000 paid 15.7 per cent of its income in health care expenditures; families with income from $3500 to $5000 paid 6.8 per cent; and those with income over $7500 paid 3.8 per cent (2). In this study health care expenditures include out-of-pocket payments and health insurance premiums, but not taxes. With the exception of the very poor, who may have been helped by Medicare and Medicaid, there is no reason to expect that this picture has changed since 1963.

Clearly, health care costs have a far lesser impact on higher income people than on poor and working-class people. This is due to the fundamentally unjust character of the two major ways in which health care has been financed: out-of-pocket payments and private health insurance premiums. Out-of-pocket payments are harder on low-income people: a $50 or $100 charge for a doctor visit, plus laboratory work and x-rays, is a catastrophe for the poor, a hardship for working-class people, and only a slight annoyance for the rich.

But many people fail to recognize the unfair nature of private health insurance payments. A family earning $6,000 might have a Blue Cross policy costing $300 per year—5 per cent of the family income. A family earning $15,000 with the same policy pays only 2 per cent of its income. This problem is compounded by the fact that poorer people may be unable to obtain group health insurance and therefore must pay higher rates for individual policies, and that poorer people who may be older or sicker are charged higher rates because they are greater risks for insurance companies.

Are tax-supported health services a more equitable method of financing health care? Thirty-seven per cent of personal health expenditures are government financed at the federal level through Medicare, Medicaid, and other programs, at the state level particularly through Medicaid and mental health expenditures and in local areas through support of public hospitals and health departments.

To address the problem of equity in government health care financing, the entire tax structure of the country must be examined. Taxes can be classified as regressive, proportional, or progressive according to how they are shared by different income groups. A regressive tax hits the poor harder than the rich. If families with income under $5,000 pay 10 per cent of that income in a certain tax while families over $15,000 pay 5 per cent of their income in the same tax, then that tax is regressive. A tax is proportional if everyone is taxed at the same percentage of his or her income, i.e. a 10 per cent across-the-board tax. A progressive tax, for example, would require rich people to pay 40 per cent of their income while poor people might pay 1 per cent.

Equitable taxation requires that people pay according to their ability. Rich people save a sizeable portion of their income, and thus, a 50 per cent tax would not cut into the amount of necessities they can afford. For poor people who spend all of their income on food, shelter, clothing, and transportation, even a 5 per cent tax presents an enormous burden. Thus proportional taxation—such as a 10 per cent tax for everyone—is not just; it hits the poor family very hard yet is of little consequence to the rich. Only progressive taxation, with a substantial increase in tax rate as income rises, is truly equitable.

THE INCOME TAX

The individual income tax accounts for 41 per cent of all tax revenues. The greatest amount of income tax revenue—$90 billion in 1970—is paid to the federal government. It is generally believed that this tax is truly progressive with the rich paying significantly more than the poor. This belief is a myth. In fact, most people pay at approximately the same tax rate. The super-rich frequently pay very little.

The income tax is not truly progressive because it rests upon a simple principle: some incomes are more taxable than others. Wages are taxed fully, income from stocks and other investments are taxed less, and income from municipal bonds are not taxed at all. Stern (3) gives the following examples: "Albert's $7,000 was earned over a year's time in a steel mill. Albert pays $1,282 in taxes. . . . Charles merely picked up the telephone, told his broker to sell some stock, and netted a $7,000 profit. Charles' tax: $526. Mrs. Horace Dodge, with $1.5 million in yearly income from municipal bonds, paid no taxes at all." These injustices invariably hurt working people who make most of their income from wages.

How does the income tax really affect people of different incomes? According to the AFL-CIO Research Department, people who earn less than $5,000 pay an average tax of 15 per cent, those with incomes from $5,000 to $10,000 pay 16 per cent, and those who earn from $10,000 to $20,000 pay an average of 18 per cent. In 1967, 76 per cent of income was subject to the 14-19 per cent rate. Most people, then, are paying taxes at essentially the same rate.

Brookings Institution economist Joseph Pechman (4) contends that rates rise from 23.5 per cent on incomes from $50,000 to $75,000 to 34 per cent on incomes over $1 million. However, he fails to take into account that a large portion of capital gains to the rich are never reported as income. Thus the actual average tax rate for those earning over $50,000 is closer to 20 per cent (5).

The federal income tax is progressive to a very slight degree. Many wealthy people take advantage of enormous tax loopholes to pay little or no tax. In 1969, 56 people with incomes over $1 million paid no federal income tax at all (6). The total amount of revenue lost to the federal government through loopholes to the rich amounts to a staggering $50 billion per year (7).

SOCIAL SECURITY

Social security payments in 1969 amounted to $44 billion in federal revenue. In describing social security, a tax expert from Brookings Institution writes, "The payroll tax is the most burdensome tax levied by the federal government on the poor in the United States" (8). A family earning from $3,000 to $4,000 pays an average of 11.3 per cent of its income in social security. Those earning from $7,500 to $10,000 pay 4.2 per cent. On incomes above $15,000 the tax is less than 1 per cent (9).

Why is social security so regressive? First, it taxes only wages. Low-income people earn money only from wages, all of which is subject to the payroll tax. People with higher incomes may have non-wage sources of money which are not taxed. Second, there is a cutoff point at $9000. A person who earns $9000 might pay $450 in social security taxes while another who makes $18,000 also pays $450. Wages above $9000 are not taxed. The first person pays a 5 per cent tax whereas the second pays only 2.5 per cent. Third, the employer's portion of social security is actually paid by the employee. Social security deducts a certain percentage of the employee's income, and also deducts money from the employer for each person on the payroll. However, the employer does not really pay his or her share, but shifts his or her portion of the payroll tax to the employee by keeping wages down. According to the Brookings Institution, most economists believe that "a major share of a payroll tax is borne by the wage earner, and some believe that all of it rests on him. . . . While they [employers] very likely are unable to reduce wages immediately after imposition of the tax, they can do so effectively over time by not increasing wages so much as they would have if the tax had not been introduced" (8). Thus the employer does not pay social security taxes. Usually the worker is taxed by receiving lower wages, and occasionally the consumer bears the burden through higher prices.

OTHER TAXES

Sales taxes brought in $39 billion in 1969, accounting for 47 per cent of revenue to state governments. These taxes hit people in proportion to the percentage of their income spent on the taxed items. A sales tax on bread or milk is extremely regressive since everyone must buy basic foods, and for the poor, food is a high proportion of the family budget. A sales tax on caviar, French champagne, or diamond rings is not regressive since poor people avoid such items. Some state sales taxes are approximately proportional since food, gas, and electricity are not taxed. Any proportional tax is not equitable since the poor are less able to afford the payments. Other states, however, place a sales tax on all items, resulting in very regressive taxation.

Even more unjust is the property tax. Although this levy accounts for only 11 per cent of all taxes, it becomes very important for local government, bringing in 40 per cent of revenue. Almost all property taxes are paid by tenants and homeowners. The property tax on business establishments is generally assessed far lower than the real value of the property and can be shifted to consumers. The property tax on apartment buildings is totally shifted to tenants in the form of higher rents. The extraordinary regressiveness of the property tax is shown by figures from Rostvold's study of California financing (10): Families earning $1,000 per year pay 13 per cent of their income in property taxes; those making from $4,000 to $5,000 pay 5 per cent in property taxes; and families with incomes above $15,000 pay only 2 per cent in property taxes.

The final major revenue producer is the corporate tax, which accounts for 15 per cent of total tax revenue, the greatest amount of which is paid to the federal government. The federal corporate tax revenue in 1969 was $39 billion. Corporate profits before taxes amounted to $136 billion. Thus the corporations appear to be taxed at the rate of 29 per cent. However, economists generally believe that corporate stockholders do not pay the entire tax themselves. As in the case of social security, corporations shift part of the tax to workers by keeping wages down, and part to consumers by raising prices. Thus only a portion of the corporate tax actually results in lowered profits. The exact percentage of corporate taxes that are shifted is not known but the figure can be estimated to be about 50 per cent. Corporations, then, are taxed at a rate closer to 15 per cent than to 29 per cent.

Some corporations find ways to avoid the corporate tax. Oil companies are a good example. In 1967, Texaco was taxed at 1.9 per cent of its income, Standard Oil of California at 1.2 per cent, and Atlantic-Richmond paid no tax at all. In 1971, McDonnell Douglas, Gulf and Western, Alcoa, and Continental Oil paid no corporate taxes. Between 1960 and 1968, corporate profits increased 91 per cent whereas corporate taxes dropped by $5 billion (7).

OVERALL TAXATION

What is the overall effect of taxation in America? As Table 1 shows, taxes hit the poor far harder than the rich (11). Taxation on incomes of up to $10,000 is actually regressive. From $10,000 to $50,000 the rate is essentially proportional. Only the very rich appear to pay a higher rate. However, the 45 per cent figure may greatly exceed the actual rate paid because of large amounts of unreported capital gains income (5). In any case, the very rich pay at a lower rate than the very poor.

Table 1
Overall tax rates, 1969

Money Income Levels	Overall Tax Rate
	%
Under $ 2,000	50.0
$ 2,000– 3,999	34.6
$ 4,000– 5,999	31.0
$ 6,000– 7,999	30.1
$ 8,000– 9,999	29.2
$10,000–14,999	29.8
$15,000–24,000	30.0
$25,000–49,999	32.8
Over $50,000	45.0

NATIONAL HEALTH INSURANCE

Two major mechanisms have been proposed for financing national health insurance—payroll deductions and general federal revenues. With the exception of the Health Security Act, which would derive 50 per cent of its income from general revenues, most congressional national health insurance proposals rely principally upon the payroll deduction.

Payroll deductions in national health insurance proposals are either compulsory employer-employee payments to private insurance companies or traditional social security. The Nixon Administration's National Health Insurance Partnership Act of 1971, the American Hospital Association's proposal, and the 1973 report of the prestigious Committee for Economic Development (12) would use employer-employee payments to private insurance companies as the basis for national health insurance programs, thus bypassing government insurance altogether for a substantial portion of the population. Employer-employee payments to insurance companies and social security are equally regressive. The average family might pay $400 in premiums per year with the employer supposedly contributing 75 per cent. However, as with social security, employers shift their portions of these payments to the employee by paying lower wages. Assuming that the entire portion of the $400 premium is paid by the employee, families with wages of $6,000 pay 6.7 per cent of this income in health insurance premiums; families earning $8,000 in wages pay 5 per cent, those making $12,000 pay 3.3 per cent; and those with wages of $20,000 pay 2 per cent. The premiums are actually more regressive than these figures show since richer people also receive income from non-wage sources which do not contribute to health insurance. In addition, these plans leave large out-of-pocket payments to the patient in the form of co-insurance, deductibles, and uncovered services. These payments are also regressive.

Under most national health insurance proposals, health insurance for the elderly would continue to be financed by social security, as would a major part of the Health Security Act and Senator Long's Catastrophic Health Insurance Program. Thus, with the exception of one-half of the Health Security Act and those portions of other national health insurance plans that finance medical care for the poor, national health insurance retains the regressive payroll deduction method of financing.

WHO PROFITS FROM PUBLIC PROGRAMS?

A sizeable portion of the federal budget is spent to help private corporations to increase their profits. These corporate subsidies well exceed $30 billion per year according to a 1971 Associated Press survey (13). The exact amount of these subsidies depends upon the definition of subsidy employed. The $30 billion figure refers to payments giving special advantages to business. If one includes all monies passing from the government to private industry, the figure is much higher.

A significant portion of the $80 billion defense budget is paid to private corporations. Twenty billion dollars are spent on procurement of supplies—buying bombs, tanks, and planes from private companies. Defense research and development costs $7 billion, which is also paid largely to private business.

Research and development is an important government subsidy. In 1969 federal research and development expenditures exceeded $17 billion or one-tenth of the entire budget. Corporations are reluctant to spend their money for research and development which is considered an expensive and risky undertaking. Although government pays, profits deriving from newly developed products belong to the companies.

Certain sectors of the economy which are "in trouble" receive large subsidies. Agriculture received $6-9 billion in 1970. Not surprisingly, large sums of this money were paid to big corporate farms which had never been in trouble. In 1970 two huge California growers alone received $4.4 million and $3.3 million in subsidies; 400 farmers were each paid over $100,000. A recent limitation on subsidy payments is being evaded by dividing large farms into smaller sections.

The purpose of the $3-4 billion foreign aid program is not to aid foreign countries as many Americans believe. Rather it serves to aid American businesses in foreign countries. The Agency for International Development (AID) loans money to underdeveloped countries, but that money is used mostly to buy American products. If

AID finances a telephone network or potable water system in Peru, the telephone poles, wires, transformers, and water pipeline must be bought from American, not Peruvian companies. American construction firms often actually build the projects. In these and other ways, foreign aid cleverly subsidizes American business.

Pollution control is another corporate subsidy. Government pays to mop up after industries have destroyed the environment and gives financial incentives to encourage industries to stop polluting. Again, the cost of controlling pollution rests on the taxpayer rather than on the corporate polluter. Numerous other subsidies benefit the corporate rich: half a billion dollars to the shipping industry, millions for airlines and railroads, government training programs for corporate employees, loan guarantees, construction contracts, and so on.

In these and countless other ways, government helps private corporations to lower their costs and to maximize their profits. Higher profits result in increased dividends for stockholders. These dividends do not go to average Americans. The richest 1.6 per cent of the population owns over 80 per cent of the stock (14). Corporate subsidies benefit the very rich almost exclusively.

National health insurance would be a new source of corporate subsidies. Presently, profits earned from financing and delivering health care amount to several billion dollars each year (15). Drug companies earn about $600 million in profits, medical supply companies make $400 million, nursing homes and proprietary hospitals earn about $150 million, and doctors receive excessive incomes compared to the earnings of other highly trained professionals such as lawyers and university professors. The profits of health insurance companies are unknown but clearly run into hundreds of millions. In addition, vast amounts are spent for profit-creating advertising: $1.5 billion per year by drug companies and unknown millions by insurance companies.

Money collected under national health insurance will be paid to these profit-makers, and will certainly increase the profits earned. Just as federal defense appropriations subsidize the military-industrial complex, national health insurance will supply the medical-industrial complex with ample profits.

WEALTH AND HEALTH

The American tax and subsidy system is not simply unjust—it is destructive to people's lives and health. Taxes, coupled with the system of corporate subsidies, transfer money from the poor to the rich, and thus are an important mechanism for perpetuating poverty in America. Poverty is the country's most important cause of death, disease, and disability.

The mortality rate for poor families is far higher than the rate for the non-poor. The number of days of disability and of injury-caused work loss is two to three times higher for the poor. Poor people have three times the amount of heart disease, four times the number of maternal deaths at childbirth, six times the amount of visual impairment, six times the number of cases of high blood pressure, and seven times the amount of arthritis than non-poor people. Infant mortality, mental illness, cancer of the cervix, tuberculosis, strokes, measles, and venereal disease occur with much greater frequency in poor areas. The poor tend to suffer from cancer of the mouth, esophagus, stomach, and lung at earlier ages than the non-poor. In New York City alone, 13,000 deaths can be linked directly with poverty each year, and many more people are needlessly disabled as a result of poverty (16).

The maldistribution of income and wealth perpetuated by the tax and subsidy system is responsible for tens of thousands of deaths in the United States each year. The creation of a progressive tax structure and the elimination of public subsidies to the rich would—far more than any national health insurance scheme—serve to restore the health of the country.

National health insurance, as a part of the unjust tax and subsidy system, actually contributes to poverty, death, and disease. National health insurance has an inherent contradiction. It purports to improve health, yet it finances health services through a tax and subsidy structure that perpetuates the illnesses of poverty. Health care financing makes sense only if it is based on progressive taxes and if it eliminates profitable subsidies to the rich.

REFERENCES

1. *The American Distribution of Income: A Structural Problem.* Study for the Joint Economic Committee of the U.S. Congress. U.S. Government Printing Office, Washington, D. C., 1972.
2. Andersen, R., and Anderson, O. *A Decade of Health Services*, p. 56. University of Chicago Press, Chicago, 1967.
3. Stern, P. *The Great Treasury Raid.* Random House, New York, 1964.
4. Pechman, J. *Federal Tax Policy.* Brookings Institution, Washington, D.C., 1971.
5. Gurley, J. G. Federal tax policy. *National Tax Journal* 20: 319-327, September 1967.
6. TRB from Washington. *New Republic* 164: 4, April 10, 1971.
7. House Ways and Means Committee. *Tax Reform, 1969*, pp. 1788, 4149, 4199, 4315. U.S. Government Printing Office, Washington, D.C., 1969.
8. Pechman, J., et al. *Social Security: Perspectives for Reform*, pp. 175, 177, 221. Brookings Institution, Washington, D.C., 1968.
9. Lampman, R. Transfer and redistribution as social process. In *Social Security in International Perspective*, edited by S. Jenkins, Columbia University Press, New York, 1969
10. Rostvold, G. *Financing California Government*. Dickenson Publishing Company, Belmont, California, 1967.
11. Herriot, R., and Miller, H. The taxes we pay. *The Conference Board Record* May 1971.
12. Committee for Economic Development, Building a National Health-Care System. April 1973.
13. *San Francisco Chronicle*, p. 5, August 1, 1971.
14. Lundborg, F. *The Rich and the Superrich*, p. 13. Bantam Books, New York, 1968.
15. The Medical Industrial Complex. *Health-PAC Bulletin* November 1969.
16. James, G. Poverty as an obstacle to health progress in our cities. *Am. J. Public Health* 55: 1757-1771, November 1965.

CHAPTER 5

Capitalizing on Illness:
The Health Insurance Industry

Thomas Bodenheimer, Steven Cummings,
and Elizabeth Harding

For an insurance company, illness is not a frightening and uncomfortable experience, it is a golden opportunity. And today, when people are willing to spend a great deal of money to avoid possible financial ruin through illness, payment for health care at the time of illness is gradually being replaced by the mass financing of private health insurance: regular collection of small amounts of money from everyone to pay for the care of people who are sick. The questions then remain: How much money is collected and from whom? What types of institutions receive and pay out the money? How much is paid out and to whom?

It is our contention in this article that private health insurance institutions have taken the progressive concept of mass financing and have used it for their own benefit and that of the health care providers. They are indeed capitalizing on people's illness.

HISTORY OF PRIVATE HEALTH INSURANCE

Two major types of private health insurance institutions exist in the United States today: the "nonprofit" tax-exempt Blue Cross and Blue Shield, and the commercial insurance companies. Although commercial insurance companies had begun to insure people against sickness in the 19th century, private health insurance only became a major industry during the Depression. At that time people had little money to pay for hospital

This chapter is a revised and updated version of Chapter 7 of *Billions for Band-Aids. An Analysis of the U.S. Health Care System and of Proposals for Its Reform* by the same authors (Medical Committee for Human Rights, P.O. Box 7677, San Francisco, California 94119, $2.25).

services, which created financial trouble for the hospitals, with empty beds and unpaid bills. As a result, hospitals joined together to organize a system of prepayment plans called Blue Cross, to which patients paid a certain amount each month, and Blue Cross paid their hospital bills.

Blue Cross has since grown immensely, and it is now the largest health insurer, with 75 local plans handling hospital insurance for 80 million private subscribers and over 20 million Medicare and Medicaid enrollees. Today, half of all the income of U.S. hospitals comes from Blue Cross, and over $12 billion passes through this giant annually.

Blue Shield also began during the Depression, when doctors noticed that many people were too poor to seek care and that those patients who did often could not pay. State medical associations sponsored the Blue Shield plans, to which patients would pay monthly sums so that Blue Shield could reimburse doctors for services. Blue Shield has also grown; its 72 local plans now insure 65 million people for medical and surgical care, and it handles 13 million Medicare and Medicaid patients.

Commercial insurance companies did not become important in the health field until after World War II, when the Blues were already well established. Labor unions, as part of their negotiations with management over wages, began to demand health benefits for workers and as these benefits were fought for and won, employers started to pay part of employees' wages into health and welfare funds, which were used to buy private health insurance at group rates.

Commercial companies were successful in capturing a large share of the union health insurance market because of the way they can set premium rates. They have a choice of setting the amount of premium by either community rating or experience rating, the first being to charge the entire population one rate, and the latter to charge a lower rate to healthier people. Under community rating, the system traditionally used by the Blues, sick people were subsidized by well people, while experience rating actually allowed insurance companies to appear benevolent to healthy people, by enabling them to charge less. Thus, commercial companies offered better deals to young, healthy workers than the Blues could offer them. And partly because they were able to obtain so much of the labor union population, commercial companies grew enormously during the 1950s. As a block, they now sell slightly more health insurance than the Blues.

Aware that experience rating allowed commercial companies to insure healthy workers more cheaply than they could, the Blues also began experience rating. This meant that older, sicker people had to pay very high rates, or were unable to be insured at all. It also implied a loss of business for the Blues. However, when Medicare, a government insurance program for the elderly, was passed in 1965, the insurance companies found a scheme for cashing in on the sickness of the elderly. In helping to write Medicare, they were able to make themselves "intermediaries" for Medicare, accepting money in the form of social security and taxes collected by government and distributing it to the providers of health care. And because of its success with Medicare, the private insurance industry has lent its support to the concept of national health insurance as long as the funds would be channeled through them.

WHAT PEOPLE GET FROM HEALTH INSURANCE

About 160 million Americans presently hold private health insurance policies. Many buy the insurance as part of a group such as a company, union, or professional organization, with their premiums often being deducted automatically from their paychecks. About 40 million have the far more expensive individual health insurance, and these people tend to be employees without access to a group, the unemployed, the self-employed and sporadically employed, and the elderly or sick.

Many insurance policies will not insure or will only partially insure the ill. Blue Cross states in one policy, "If at the time your application is reviewed a condition is found which excludes you from enrollment, you may be given an opportunity to join with a waiver for that condition." In other words, if you are sick, you can buy our policy and your medical expenses will be covered, but only if you get a different illness.

The elderly, under experience rating, pay more for health insurance. A Prudential policy offering hospital coverage costs $318.36 per year for a 26-year-old female and $482.36 for a 58-year-old female. Women are generally charged more than men for the same coverage because they use medical care more frequently. And people with chronic illness such as high blood pressure or diabetes must pay more for insurance, if they can obtain insurance at all.

All types of health insurance have deductibles and uncovered or partially covered care. Deductibles refer to the amount the consumer must pay for services before the insurance company will pay. Medicare patients are required to pay the first $84 of their hospital bill and the first $60 a year of their doctors' bills. A major medical plan offered by Connecticut General begins paying for covered services after the consumer has paid a $750 deductible. A similar plan by Prudential has a $400 deductible, and Equitable offers major medical plans with from $500 to $2000 deductibles.

Insurance companies generally make patients pay part of the costs of services. Partially covered care is expressed in two ways: the first is called co-insurance—we pay 80 per cent and you pay 20 per cent; the second is limited coverage—we pay for 60 days of care, you pay the rest. Insurance salesmen call this "sharing the risk with us." Medicare requires patients to pay $21 per day of their hospital bill for the 61st to 90th hospital day, $10.50 per day for the 21st to 100th nursing home day, and 20 per cent of the bill for visits to the doctor. A group Blue Cross plan requires the policyholder to pay 20 per cent for almost all services received outside the hospital, and 20 per cent of the hospital bill after 70 days; the plan pays only $100 for outpatient psychiatric care. Innumerable additional examples could be listed.

Every insurance policy leaves many medical services uncovered. The best examples of such services are dental care, outpatient psychiatric care, preventive care, and outpatient drugs. Medicare fails to pay for eye and hearing examinations, glasses or hearing aids, routine checkups, and outpatient drugs. A Connecticut General major medical insurance policy pays for no outpatient care at all. A group basic benefit plan offered by Equitable pays for no visits to doctors' offices, no psychiatric care, no dental care, and no outpatient drugs.

About 20 per cent of the population has no private surgical and hospital insurance, 28 per cent has no in-the-hospital physician insurance, 55 per cent has no insurance for physician visits, 48 per cent has no insurance for prescribed drugs, and 93 per cent has no dental insurance (1).

An average family of four has the following medical needs: yearly physical examinations by a doctor for all members, four visits to the doctor for illness, a yearly dental checkup and needed dental work. prescription drugs for three members, and an eye examination and glasses for one member. The standard insurance policy will pay for none of these services and costs the family about $350 per year.

Private insurance advocates claim that deductibles, uncovered, and partially covered care prevent the consumer from "overusing" health facilities. In reality, however, two studies show that out-of-pocket payments mainly prevent lower-income people from using needed services (2). With the average person covered for only 42 per cent of health costs (1), and with these costs rising each year, out-of-pocket expenses even for insured middle-class people can be financially disastrous as the following examples show (3):

- In 1969 the daughter of two federal government employees had a sudden attack of intestinal disease with complications in the liver and lungs. She was hospitalized for 44 days, with a bill of $7571. Even with her parents' comparatively good insurance, the family had to pay $1550 out-of-pocket.
- In 1965 an engineer was stricken with kidney disease. In three months he ran up medical bills of $24,000. His Blue Cross and Blue Shield policies left $9000 unpaid. The patient lost his $3000 in savings, sold his car and some furniture, moved to a small apartment, and went on welfare.

WHO CONTROLS AND PROFITS FROM PRIVATE HEALTH INSURANCE?

Blue Cross

Local Blue Cross plans have always been dominated by representatives of the hospitals. Fifty per cent of Blue Cross board members throughout the country have been hospital administrators and trustees (4). Other Blue Cross directors are often doctors and businessmen with hospital ties. In 1969, for example, the Massachusetts Blue Cross 31-member board had 11 trustees who were representatives of hospitals, 9 trustees from corporations with close hospital ties, and 4 doctors who were important individuals in hospitals. The other 7 members represented business and labor.

What is the effect of hospital domination of Blue Cross boards? Because of hospital control, Blue Cross has tended to channel as much money as possible to hospitals. This is done by the "cost plus" method of reimbursement. Essentially, Blue Cross has paid anything and everything that the hospital has asked for.

It is impossible to determine exactly how much a hospital should be paid for each patient. Does the payment include the cost of running an underutilized, unnecessary open-heart surgery unit even though the patient didn't use that unit? The cost of paying interest on a loan for building a half-empty hospital wing? The cost of hiring labor-relations consultants to stop the employees from organizing unions? The cost of the hospital's public relations budget? The cost of educational and training programs for nurses or interns? The cost of large increases in administrative salaries?

Blue Cross pays all these things, "negotiating" with hospitals every year or two about exactly which costs it will reimburse. Only occasionally will Blue Cross refuse to pay for certain items. Thus Blue Cross has allowed hospitals to continue to raise rates without questioning the reasons for the increases. Only one-fifth of Blue Cross plans make audits of hospital accounts (4). If Blue Cross used its power, it could change the practices of hospitals. In New York City, for example, Blue Cross pays for over two-thirds of hospital costs; with such leverage, Blue Cross could easily force hospitals to control unnecessary costs (5).

However, Blue Cross cannot be seen as simply a collection agency for hospitals. Another set of interests impinges on the hospitals' control over Blue Cross. Any institution channeling billions of dollars a year is a prime target for conflict of interest, and Blue Cross is no exception.

Between 1968 and 1970, the Richmond, Virginia, Blue Cross paid a highly excessive $1.2 million for furniture bought from a company, one of whose officials was a director of Blue Cross. The same Blue Cross plan paid an inflated $200,000 to a data processing company that had a member on its board. Board members may also use their position for petty personal gain; Virginia Blue Cross executives drove in company cars to a distant resort and charged Blue Cross for first-class air fare (6).

In the 1960s, the Washington, D.C., Blue Cross deposited between $10 and $20 million over a six-year period in bank accounts that paid no interest to Blue Cross. There is no reason to keep large non-interest-bearing accounts. Most of this money was deposited in the National Savings and Trust Company, and the bank profited $800,000 a year by not paying interest to Blue Cross. Blue Cross' board chairman was a board member of National Savings and Trust, and the bank's president was the Blue Cross treasurer who makes Blue Cross' investment decisions (7).

Shortly after the Vice President of Continental Illinois National Bank became chairman of Illinois Blue Cross, Blue Cross' bank deposit jumped to $7 million, with not one cent of interest for Blue Cross. The yearly interest of $400,000 could have paid the 8-day hospital bills of 500 Blue Cross subscribers. The Northern Trust Company, with another Illinois Blue Cross board member, pays no interest on $2 million in Blue Cross deposits (8). These examples show how a so-called nonprofit institution (Blue Cross) can be used to make profits for the companies run by Blue Cross trustees.

Blue Cross has also built beautiful buildings for itself, pays high salaries (Walter McNerney, head of the Blue Cross Association that coordinates the 75 local plans, has a salary of $80,000), and it constantly attempts to bring in more money than it spends. And Blue Cross' administrative expenses have inflated at a rapid rate; between 1965 and 1969 the administrative costs for all local Blue Cross plans increased 66.2 per cent (9).

Blue Cross, then, operates more and more like a profit-making institution. It may have smaller profits than other corporations, and these profits are used for growth, reserves, and conflict-of-interest rather than for dividends to stockholders, but, all the same, the concept of paying out as little as possible is coming to dominate the operation of Blue Cross. Naturally, this "profit-making" concept is at odds with the concept of a "hospital collection agency." In the latter case, as much as possible of Blue Cross' funds are channeled to hospitals. In the former, Blue Cross tries to limit payment to hospitals in order to have more for administrative salaries, bank and furniture "rip-offs," and growth. Below we will explore some of these conflicts within Blue Cross.

Who, then, profits from Blue Cross? Most of all, health providers and suppliers: profit-making hospitals; hospital supply companies that sell to hospitals; and construction companies whose structures are paid for by loans from insurance companies and banks, with Blue Cross paying the interest. Secondly, the banks and furniture companies that channel profits from Blue Cross' administrative expenses. And thirdly, Blue Cross itself, whose executives pay themselves well and whose net income is used for expansion through advertising and promotion.

Expansion is a key issue for Blue Cross, particularly with national health insurance on the drawing board. A September 10, 1971, memo from Walter McNerney to all local Blue Cross plans revealed a confidential plan for extensive Congressional lobbying to make Blue Cross central to any legislative health care reforms. In the words of Health/PAC,

Blue Cross is "shining its shoes and combing its hair, ready to step forward as the prime candidate for intermediary or administrative agent for national health insurance (10).

Blue Shield

Blue Shield usually covers doctors' visits and surgery while Blue Cross takes care of hospital costs. Blue Shield belongs to the doctors, with most local Blue Shield plans controlled by local or state medical societies. In 1970, about two-thirds of all Blue Shield board members were doctors. The governing board of California Blue Shield, for example, is composed of 21 members. Nineteen are physicians chosen by the California Medical Association; the other two are "consumers," also elected by the California Medical Association. The current two "consumers" on the board are the regional president of the Bank of America and the personnel director of General Motors.

The way in which Blue Shield protects doctors' fees can be seen from the method of reimbursement. Blue Shield generally pays doctors the "usual and customary" fee. This fee, which is an average of the fees of all doctors in a geographic area, can be raised by the doctors themselves. Sometimes individual doctors raise their fees; often local medical societies decide that doctors' fees should be raised for the whole county. From 1966 through 1971, doctors have annually raised their usual and customary fees by 7 per cent per year (7.5 per cent in 1970-1971) (11). When Blue Shield makes a contract with a doctor, that doctor is generally not allowed to charge patients above what Blue Shield pays the doctor. However, many doctors do not participate in Blue Shield; they can charge their patients their standard fee, and Blue Shield will reimburse the patient for part of the fee.

Thus Blue Shield allows the doctor to be in the most advantageous position imaginable. Doctors set their own usual and customary fees. But if the fee is not enough for a particular doctor, he or she can charge the patient more, and Blue Shield will pay part. The consumer has no control over the amount the doctor is paid.

Blue Shield, then, primarily profits the private physician. However, Blue Shield is not free from exploitation by banks, corporations, and Blue Shield executives. Eleven per cent of Blue Shield's $3 billion income (not including government programs) is used for administrative expenses (9). This creates a quarter of a billion dollars for high salaries, new buildings, advertising, and profitable subcontracts (see below).

Commercial Insurance Companies

Unlike the Blues, which were put together to assure the payment of bills to the hospitals and doctors, commercial insurance companies sell health insurance purely for the purpose of making a profit. About 1000 companies offer health insurance, with about 115 million people holding some type of commercial policy. In 1972, the commercials took in $14.3 billion in premium income (12). Thus the total volume of commercial insurance is somewhat greater than that of the Blues, though no one commercial company comes close to Blue Cross in size.

The ten largest commercial health insurers are Aetna, Travelers, Metropolitan Life, Prudential, CNA, Equitable, Mutual of Omaha, Connecticut General, John Hancock, and Provident. In 1970, Aetna took in over a billion dollars in health premiums (13).

Most of the top health insurance companies are also the biggest life insurers. These giants represent an enormous concentration of wealth and political power in America. Prudential and Metropolitan Life, the two largest, each have $30 billion in assets, making them far bigger than General Motors, Standard Oil of New Jersey, and ITT, and the equals of Bank of America and Chase Manhattan Bank. In 1970, supposedly a bad year for health insurance, the life insurance business boomed. In that year Prudential and Metropolitan Life received premium income (life, accident, health, and other policies) of almost $4 billion each and net income from investments of $1.4 billion each (13).

The major insurance companies are closely tied to the largest U.S. banks and manufacturing corporations through enormous financial empires. The Rockefeller family interests control or heavily influence the Metropolitan Life and Equitable insurance companies, Chase Manhattan Bank, Standard Oil, Mobil Oil, IBM, and numerous other corporations. The Morgan empire (the legacy of J. P. Morgan) includes the Prudential Insurance Company, the Bankers Trust and Morgan Guarantee Trust banks, General Electric, and U.S. Steel. Of 28 directors of Metropolitan Life, 23 sit on the boards of banking institutions, particularly Chase Manhattan. Eighteen of Prudential's 29 directors sit on bank boards. Half of Equitable's directors are on bank boards with an especially close relation with Chase Manhattan (14).

These facts are given in order to make the point that commercial health insurance policy is ultimately set by very rich and influential people in U.S. society. The money that comes into the hands of these companies, constituting one-half of the net savings of individuals in America (15), is used in several ways: (a) to make huge loans ($185 million daily) to corporations, thus supplying much of the money needed for corporate expansion; (b) to buy large blocks of stock in corporations so that the insurance company can effectively control the corporations; (c) to finance real estate developments and urban high-rise buildings; and (d) to influence politicians through campaign contributions and other favors (for example, W. Clement Stone, chairman of Combined Insurance, the thirteenth largest health insurer, gave $1 million to Richard Nixon's 1968 campaign, another million to the 1972 campaign, and received a preferential ruling from the Price Commission in 1971 to raise insurance rates) (16).

Commercial insurance companies have a different relationship with doctors and hospitals than do the Blues. Whereas the Blues make contracts with hospitals and doctors regarding how much they will pay, a commercial company contracts with the patient and does not deal with the providers directly. Thus patients often have to fight to collect the money from their insurance company.

Commercial companies formerly paid the patient only a stipulated sum of money for each service, for example, $50 per hospital day despite the fact that the daily charge might be $80. Many individual policies are still written this way. One plan advertized in a San Francisco newspaper pays $100 per week ($14.28 per day) for hospital care while hospital rates are around $100 per day. The advertisement contained the sentence: "When hospital emergency strikes, you can say 'Thank Heaven, we didn't have to borrow a cent.'"

However, commercial group plans have generally changed due to competition among themselves and with the Blues. Many of these plans now pay the full daily hospital rate, though with the usual deductibles, co-insurance, and limitations. Commercials thus have become concerned with the rapid rise in hospital charges since they too must pay out more when the rates go up.

In 1972, commercial companies collected $14.3 billion in insurance premiums and paid out $10.6 billion in benefit payments (12). On the average, group policies pay out in benefits 96 per cent of the premiums collected, whereas individual policies pay out only 51 per cent. Clearly, individual plans pay far fewer benefits and thus are of less value to the buyer than are group plans (17). Different companies pay out higher or lower percentages of their premium income depending on whether they have more or less group coverage. In 1970, Aetna and Travelers paid out 90 per cent of their premium income; these companies overwhelmingly sell group insurance. Metropolitan Life and Prudential paid out around 85 per cent of premiums, whereas Mutual of Omaha paid only 73 per cent and Combined Insurance (run by former President Nixon's friend W. Clement Stone) paid out only 43 per cent of its largely individual premiums (13).

In light of the profit orientation of insurance companies, it may come as a surprise that in 1970, the commercial insurance industry spent $600 million more in benefits and administrative costs than it collected in premiums. Aetna, the largest commercial insurer, collected $1 billion in 1970 premiums, paid out $984 million in benefits, spent millions more in administration, and consequently lost $13 million on its health insurance. In 1969 Aetna lost $28 million on health insurance; in 1968, $16 million; and in 1967 it gained $6 million. In 1970 Travelers lost $41 million in health insurance; Metropolitan Life lost $18 million; Connecticut General lost $37 million; and Combined Insurance gained $16 million (13). By 1972, however, the companies as a whole were doing better, as we will describe later.

Are health insurance companies really losing money? The answer is no. First, commercial health insurance is closely linked to life and other forms of insurance. A large amount of group commercial insurance (perhaps $2-3 billion a year) is bought by companies who pay for workmen's compensation, disability, life, accident, and health insurance for their employees. These companies generally study the policies of several insurers and buy all the insurance in a package from one insurance company. Thus, an insurance company that makes a good offer on health insurance will sell more of the highly profitable life insurance, and the apparent health insurance losses are actually bringing in greater profits in other types of insurance.

Secondly, the health insurance losses do not take investment income into account. When Aetna collects $1 billion in health insurance premiums, it does not pay this money out in benefits right away. The money is available for investment, which produces a profitable return. Aetna's total investment income in 1970 was $344 million (13). Since 55 per cent of Aetna's premiums are from health insurance, one can assume that Aetna earned $190 million in investments from its health business. Thus the $13 million in "losses" is erased, and Aetna actually profited immensely from its health insurance.

MEDICARE AND MEDICAID: PUBLIC PRIVATE INSURANCE

Medicare and Medicaid were passed by Congress in 1965 as amendments to the Social Security Act. The insurance industry's role in these government programs is important to study because it provides a model for understanding the profit-making potential of national health insurance (18).

Because of high co-insurance, deductibles, partial premiums, and uncovered services, Medicare pays for only 42 per cent of the health bill of the average person over 65 years of age. In fiscal year 1972, out-of-pocket costs for the average Medicare recipient reached $404, which is $95 more than the elderly's out-of-pocket expenses in the year before Medicare began (19). This worsening situation for the elderly in spite of Medicare is caused by inflation and by major yearly increases in Medicare's deductibles, premiums, and co-insurance.

Medicaid, designed to provide access to health care for low-income people, has also fallen far short of providing for the needs of those it was established to help (20). Only half of the 40 million poor people in the United States are covered at all, and many are faced with limitations in services offered. Because Medicaid pays lower fees than private insurance, many doctors will not accept Medicaid recipients; in New York City, for example, 23 per cent of physicians treat Medicaid patients, and 4 per cent of physicians collect 85 per cent of all Medicaid fees (21).

Medicare and Medicaid are big business. In fiscal year 1972 Medicare cost $8.8 billion and Medicaid $7.6 billion. In the following discussion we will chiefly deal with Medicare; in most instances the workings of Medicaid are similar.

The Intermediaries

Under these government programs, providers of health care deal directly with intermediaries rather than with the federal or state governments. For Medicare Part A (inpatient services), hospitals and nursing homes choose the intermediaries. Blue Cross handles 93 per cent of Medicare payments to hospitals and 53 per cent to extended care facilities. Under Part B (physician services) the federal government chooses the intermediaries, 60 per cent going to Blue Shield. Under Medicaid the state government picks the intermediaries, which are also largely the Blues (22).

Within certain limits, the intermediaries determine how much to pay the providers of care. The Medicare law has allowed hospitals to be paid the reasonable costs of services, whereas doctors have received "usual and customary" fees. As with private Blue plans, the hospital and doctor decide on the amount of payment, the Blues pay up, and the government reimburses them for costs and administrative expenses.

Blue Cross pays hospitals at regular intervals during the year. At the end of the year, when the hospital's true yearly costs are calculated, the hospital can readjust its bill to Blue Cross. Can you imagine your grocer calling you at the end of the year to state that you owe $50 more because he or she did not anticipate expenses correctly?

Doctors can bill their Medicare patients, forcing the patient to collect from Blue Shield. Many Medicare patients must fill out complicated forms only to find that Blue Shield is not paying them back for the entire bill. Other doctors bill Blue Shield directly, and the patient has only the 20 per cent co-insurance to worry about.

Who Profits from Medicare and Medicaid?

Because the Blues—who represent doctors and hospitals—have gained such a grip on Medicare and Medicaid, providers of health care have been allowed to make immense profits from these programs. As has been pointed out,

> In no other realm of economic life today are payments guaranteed for costs that are neither controlled by competition nor regulated by public authority, and in which no incentives for economy can be discerned (22, p. 192).

Medicare brought an enormous inflation in health care costs. Hospital costs increased by 6.4 per cent per year from 1956-1965, and 13.4 per cent per year from 1965-1970, and the jump in inflation occurred immediately after the passage of Medicare. In 1965 the costs rose 5.8 per cent, whereas in 1967 they increased 19.0 per cent. Doctors' fees rose by 3.5 per cent annually between 1960 and 1967, and from 1967 to 1971 the yearly increase was 6.7 per cent, indicating a sudden jump at the onset of Medicare (11). On the stock market, shares for profit-making nursing homes boomed after Medicare was passed. Nonprofit hospitals increased their net income. Hospital construction soared, with the number of beds increasing at a rate three times greater than the rise in population, resulting in an overbedding crisis that now costs hospital users hundreds of millions of dollars a year (23). In California, government health expenditures for low-income people increased by 500 per cent from 1965 to 1970, with 250 per cent being due to price rises rather than to the introduction of more services for more people (24).

These increased costs and resultant profits were caused by the intermediary system. The Blues made no attempt to control costs. In many cases, the Blues paid providers for care not covered by Medicare or Medicaid. According to a Social Security Administration audit, 11 per cent of Northern California Blue Cross claims were for uncovered services. In addition, the Blues often paid fees that were more than "usual and customary." Alabama Blue Shield, for example, allowed doctors to charge their Medicare patients between 25 and 400 per cent more than ordinary Blue Shield patients (25). New York City Medicare fees may be two to three times those paid for private Blue Shield patients. Even New York Blue Shield's vice-president stated that Medicare is a "gold mine for doctors" (26).

Also, many cases have been uncovered of duplicate payments to the same provider. In 1967, California Blue Shield was estimated to have paid $350,000 per month in duplicate payments. Also through Medicare and Medicaid, providers were free to do unnecessary procedures on patients. The children of Medicaid recipients in California undergo four times as much surgery as other children in California (27).

How extensive has Medicare-Medicaid profiteering been? In 1968 at least 5000 individual practitioners were paid over $25,000 by Medicare. Several hundred earned over $100,000 per year (25). Department of Health, Education, and Welfare audits show that Colorado Blue Shield paid $2.4 million in unnecessary payments in 1968-1969. Connecticut General Insurance Company made duplicate Medicare payments of $1.2 million between 1966 and 1969. Aetna Life Insurance Company made $4.5 million in excess Medicare payments during the same period; Massachusetts Blue Shield, $1.9 million excess payments; Occidental Life Insurance Company, $3.2 million; Northern California Blue Cross, $18.6 million; Southern California Blue Cross, $14.2 million (28).

A grand jury claimed that New York Medicaid has wasted $1 billion in nursing home bills for dead patients, pharmacists charging for pills not given to patients, doctors sending patients back and forth between physicians, and other such practices (29). Some labs charged Medicaid for sickle-cell anemia tests on white patients and—in one instance, a pregnancy test on a man (30). In addition to these cases of fraud and error, the use of "usual and customary fee" and "reasonable costs" has resulted in inflation costing the Medicare and Medicaid programs hundreds of millions of dollars (25).

Health providers are not the only Medicare and Medicaid profit makers. Blue Cross and Blue Shield and their subcontractors have also made money on the programs. In fiscal year 1971, for example, Medicare administrative expenses came to about $250 million, and part of the administrative costs paid to the Blues by the government are used to pay the costs of the Blues' commercial business. Also, the Blues can collect Medicare payments from the federal government and delay their payments to providers, thus allowing themselves to collect interest on the federal money. Through this procedure California Blue Shield has gained $180.000 in interest.

One of the grossest examples of Medicare-Medicaid profiteering is the subcontracting of data processing to profit-making corporations. In fiscal year 1970, data processing costs for Medicare came to $63 million (31). Much of this work is subcontracted, which seems ironic since the Blues initially recommended themselves as fiscal intermediaries partially because of their expertise in claims processing.

Electronic Data Systems (EDS), a Texas firm run by Ross Perot, processes claims for Medicare and Medicaid in 11 states, and carries out work for some of the biggest programs. Originally, Perot worked for Texas Blue Shield, and he convinced his employer to give him a subcontract to do the data processing through EDS, which he set up. As a result, Perot has become "The Fastest Richest Texan Ever" with a personal fortune approaching $1 billion (32). One of Perot's large contracts has been for California's Medicaid program, the head of which became an EDS consultant shortly after the contract was approved. Forty-two per cent of the administrative costs of the California program go to Perot, whose profits average 40 per cent. While it costs EDS only 28 cents to process a claim, the firm charges California Blue Shield 70 cents per claim, which amount Blue Shield passes on to the government.

RECENT CHANGES IN THE HEALTH INSURANCE INDUSTRY

The enormous inflation allowed by the Blues in Medicare and Medicaid produced a serious paradox: the very organizations that had helped cause the inflation, themselves began to suffer from it. Hospital and doctor costs soared not only under Medicare and Medicaid, but in private health insurance plans as well. The Blues and commercial companies found that they were having a hard time paying out all the money the providers were demanding. In addition, the government and locally organized health consumers began to react to the mounting costs.

By 1970, cost control had become the number one item on the national health care agenda, affecting governments, consumer groups, and even the insurance industry itself. What are some examples of the cost-control movement?

- Government cuts in Medicare reimbursement. In 1969 the Social Security administration suddenly abolished the 2 per cent plus factor paid to hospitals and nursing homes. In early 1971, physician fees were limited, and in 1972 the Social Security Amendments (P.L. 92-603) restricted fees even further (33).
- Cuts in services and reimbursement under Medicaid. Practically every state announced a Medicaid crisis in 1970-1971 (34). As a result of large Medicaid budget deficits, states cut back services to the poor. In California, for instance, patients are allowed only two doctor visits and two prescriptions per month without going through a complex system of prior authorization. In 1971, 75,000 enrollees were dropped from New York Medicaid (this came after about one million people had been cut off in 1968 and 1969) (35). In addition, Medicaid programs have also cut fees, paying doctors below what they receive from private patients.
- The Nixon Administration's series of wage-price controls limited health care cost increases for both doctors and hospitals, and the resurgence of inflation following the 1974 lifting of these controls may occasion new and tougher regulation.

- Consumers are protesting Blue Cross rate increases. In a few states, public hearings can be held on these increases. In 1969 the Student Health Organization protested Blue Cross' raising of rates up to 52 per cent in Massachusetts. In 1971 a coalition of groups in Philadelphia protested a 20 per cent Blue Cross increase (that followed a 23 per cent increase in 1970) and demanded subscriber policy making in Blue Cross. In New York, Blue Cross raised its rates 43 per cent in 1970, and a subscribers' coalition protested a subsequent 19 per cent increase in 1971 (36). In 1970 the United Auto Workers protested a Michigan Blue Cross and Blue Shield rate increase and called for removal of the Blues from the control of health providers (37).
- Consumers have even challenged how the Blues spend their money. Class action suits by Colorado Blue Cross and Blue Shield subscribers have claimed that the Blues' new $28 million building is "lavish, extravagant, wasteful and uneconomical," and the suits seek to restrain the Blues from raising rates for the purpose of accumulating surplus funds. In addition, the suits charge conflict of interest by board members and state that the Blues have spent significant amounts on unneeded hospital expansion (38).
- Several state insurance commissioners are questioning the Blue Cross-hospital relationship. The best known has been Pennsylvania's Herbert Denenberg, who has caused the Blues to shake in their boots. The "Denenberg special" consisted of no rate increase without concessions, with the demanded concessions usually including the seating of consumers on boards and less padding in payments to providers (39, 40). However, the reforms actually accomplished have been minor (for example, Denenberg settled for an increase in Pennsylvania Blue Shield consumer board members from four to eight whereas his original demand was for all physicians on the board to resign). Moreover, substantial rate increases are generally granted (41).
- Blue Cross and Blue Shield are being pressured to accept more consumers on their boards. After many state Blue Cross plans increased the numbers of their consumer board members, the Blue Cross Association took the position that all local Blue Cross boards must have a majority of consumers by January 1, 1975. However, the method for choosing consumers is far from democratic, and the "consumers" are generally of the same social status as those on hospital boards, that is, businessmen and lawyers. Thirty-five per cent of Blue Shield members across the country are now members of "the public" (not doctors or hospital representatives); of these, over 70 per cent are businessmen or lawyers (42).
- Blue Cross and the hospitals are beginning to fight each other. Blue Cross plans in Massachusetts and Philadelphia are refusing to pay hospitals everything they ask for. Illinois Blue Cross is pressuring hospitals to stop making unnecessary capital improvements.
- Blue Shield and doctors are beginning to fight each other. The Oklahoma State Medical Association withdrew endorsement of Oklahoma Blue Shield in 1971 because the Blue Shield management was offering too many positions to consumers. A large group of doctors in California tried to pull the California Medical Association out of Blue Shield because Blue Shield, in order to gain back depleted reserves, was paying doctors reduced fees.
- In two instances, Blues are being removed from their roles as fiscal intermediaries in Medicare and Medicaid. In 1973, Medicare officials acted to oust Oklahoma Blue

Theodore Lownik Library
Illinois Benedictine College
Lisle, Illinois 60532

Cross because of poor performance. In 1972, the Michigan State Department of Social Services took over administration of the Medicaid program (43).

- Professional Standards Review Organizations (PSROs), mandated by the Social Security Amendments of 1972, aim to reduce unnecessary procedures by requiring physician review of Medicare and Medicaid claims. However, the unrelenting opposition by organized medicine to the PSRO law places its effective implementation in serious question.

- Health Maintenance Organizations (HMOs) are the most important cost-control mechanism because by reversing financial incentives, there will be a tendency for underutilization in contrast to the fee-for-service tendency for overutilization. HMOs are therefore a more fundamental answer to present reimbursement formulas that reward inefficiency and spur inflation.

Though the cost-control movement claims to benefit consumers at the expense of health care providers, in fact consumers—particularly low-income people—stand to lose, with the insurance industry ending up the big winner. When Medicare fees are cut, doctors may choose to bill their patients for the portion of the fee uncollectable from the fiscal intermediary. With cuts in Medicaid fees, fewer and fewer doctors are seeing Medicaid patients at all, and money-saving cuts in Medicaid services directly hurt the patient. The 1972 Social Security Amendments are now requiring partial premiums and co-insurance for some Medicaid patients.

The federal price controls on hospitals and reduced Blue Cross reimbursement can lead to tighter billing of uninsured patients and cutting back of money-losing community services. Physician response to governmental action is to punish the low-income patient: in 1972 the Pennsylvania Medical Society threatened to boycott Medicaid until Denenberg was fired (44), and the Michigan State Medical Society advised its members not to participate in Medicaid if the State takeover of the program from Blue Shield led to reimbursement problems (43).

Most importantly, HMOs are set up to control costs by controlling patients' access to medical care. The practice of a number of HMOs for Medicaid patients in Southern California demonstrates how the HMO principle can lead to dangerously low hospital utilization rates and physician-patient ratios (45). Yet at the same time, HMOs are no guarantee against inflation. For the past several years, the cost of the country's largest HMO, the Kaiser Foundation Health Plan, has risen at a rate faster than the Consumer Price Index for Medical Care (46).

In addition to adverse effects on consumers, an immediate result of the cost-control movement is a vast increase in insurance company profits. Insurers are less willing to pay out money to doctors and hospitals, and the federal price control mechanism is holding down hospital inflation more than it is limiting insurance premium rises. Thus, private health insurers doubled their administrative costs and profits between 1971 and 1973, with the increase from 1972 to 1973 being $1 billion (47, 48).

WHAT'S WRONG WITH PRIVATE HEALTH INSURANCE?

Private health insurance does great harm to the U.S. health care system for a number of reasons:

- The insurance companies siphon off billions of dollars of people's money for health care. In 1972, the insurance industry collected $25.7 billion in health premiums and paid out $21 billion in benefits (12, pp. 35, 45). Fully $4.7 billion in one year was wasted in administrative costs, high executive salaries, competitive advertizing, sales promotion, and profits. A publicly financed health system based on salaries and budgeting rather than fee-for-service and individual claims could save a large portion of this sum.

- Twenty-five million people (12 per cent of the population) are entirely without private insurance, Medicare, or Medicaid, and unable to afford needed health care (49). Many more have grossly inadequate insurance, with the result that inability to meet medical expenses is the number one cause of personal bankruptcy in the country (50).

- Insurance companies, especially the Blues, have helped to keep the cost of medical care high and rising. The Blues, in both private and public programs, have tended to pay anything hospitals and doctors asked for. Blue Cross provides over 50 per cent of hospital income, so that it does have the power to say "no" to rising hospital rates. However, although a tendency toward more cost-consciousness is beginning, by and large no major changes have occurred, and those changes that have taken place tend to make care less accessible to consumers.

- Insurance companies have helped to grossly distort medical practice, with expensive and dangerous effects. The best known distortion is the push of health insurance toward hospitalization. Many more people have hospital insurance than insurance for ambulatory care. Therefore, patients are hospitalized for minor diagnostic tests and treatment which could be done outside the hospital. It is estimated that 30 per cent of days spent in the hospital are unnecessary (51). A more significant distortion has been the push toward surgery. Many more people have surgical insurance than insurance for nonsurgical physician services. Thus the tendency of surgeons to over-operate is reinforced by the insurance structure. Two million unnecessary operations are performed in the U.S. each year, resulting in at least 10,000 needless deaths (52, 53).

CONCLUSION

Private health insurance institutions have no reason to exist in the health care system. They are presently in the health business to make money—for themselves, for doctors, and for hospitals.

The only reasonable thing to do with the health insurance industry is to abolish it. Health care can be financed by government collection of taxes and payment directly to health centers and hospitals, without profit.

But it is not enough to abolish insurance companies. The entire notion of insurance is unfair. With insurance, people get what they pay for. Sicker people pay more than healthy people; the elderly pay more than the young; and lower-income people pay the same premiums as wealthy people, thus taking a larger percentage of their earnings.

The entire philosophy of insurance is in sharp conflict with the concept of health care as a right. If health care is a right, money should not be a consideration in receiving it. Health care should be free to everybody and should be paid for by a progressive tax based on ability to pay. The insurance concept—that people receive only what they pay for—should be thrown out along with the insurance industry.

REFERENCES

1. Mueller, M. S. Private health insurance in 1971: Health care services, enrollment, and finances. *Social Security Bulletin* 36(2): 3-22, 1973.
2. Of paying and queuing. *Notes on Health Politics* 1: 1-2, September 1, 1973.
3. Hoyt, E. *Your Health Insurance: A Story of Failure.* The John Day Company, New York, 1970.
4. Ridgeway, J. Blue Cross. *Ramparts* 9(10): 4-6, 46-47, 1971.
5. Health Policy Advisory Center. *The American Health Empire: Power, Profits and Politics*, p. 155. Vintage Books, New York, 1971.
6. U.S. Senate Subcommittee on Antitrust and Monopoly. *High Cost of Hospitalization*, pp. 3-66. U.S. Government Printing Office, Washington, D.C., 1971.
7. U.S. House of Representatives Subcommittee on Intergovernmental Relations. *Administration of Federal Health Benefit Programs*, Part 2. U.S. Government Printing Office, Washington, D.C., 1970.
8. Bajonski, A. The Blue Cross double cross. *Chicago Journalism Review*, February 1972.
9. Weiss, R. J., et al. Trends in health insurance operating expenses. *N. Engl. J. Med.* 287: 638-642, 1972.
10. Kotelchuck, R. Trying to shake the Blues. *Health/PAC Bulletin*, March 1971.
11. *Medical Care Costs and Prices: Background Book.* Social Security Administration, Department of Health, Education, and Welfare, January 1972.
12. *Source Book of Health Insurance Data*, pp. 36, 43. Health Insurance Institute, New York, 1973-1974.
13. *Best's Insurance Reports, Life-Health, 1971.* A. M. Best Company, Morristown, N.J., 1971.
14. Menshikov, S. *Millionaires and Managers.* Progress Publishers, Moscow, 1969.
15. Perlo, V. *The Empire of High Finance.* International Publishers, New York, 1957.
16. Rich Nixon contributor: Price favoratism denied. *San Francisco Chronicle*, p. 6, October 6, 1972.
17. *Basic Facts on the Health Industry.* House Committee on Ways and Means, June 1971.
18. *Who Will Pay Your Bills. A Health/PAC Special Report on National Health Insurance.* Health Policy Advisory Council, San Francisco, 1973.
19. Medical burden on the aged. *San Francisco Chronicle*, p. 30. June 27, 1973.
20. Blake, E. Medicaid: The fading of a dream. *Health/PAC Bulletin*, April 1973.
21. *Congressional Record*, 119: E1450, March 12, 1973.
22. Somers, H., and Somers, A. *Medicare and the Hospitals: Issues and Prospects*, pp. 32-35. Brookings Institution, Washington, D.C., 1967.
23. Nichols, R. Oklahoma crude. *Health/PAC Bulletin*, March-April 1974.
24. Gartside, F. Causes of increase in Medicaid costs in California. *Health Services Reports* 88: 225-235, 1973.
25. U.S. Senate Finance Committee. *Medicare and Medicaid. Problems, Issues and Alternatives.* U.S. Government Printing Office, Washington, D.C., 1970.
26. The Manhattan doctor: Medicare fees aren't hurting his health. *New York Times*, p. E4, November 25, 1973.
27. U.S. Senate Finance Committee. *National Health Insurance*, p. 36. U.S. Government Printing Office, Washington, D.C., 1971.
28. Millions wasted over Medicare. *San Francisco Examiner*, p. 6, March 7, 1972.
29. A big Medicaid scandal in N.Y. *San Francisco Chronicle*, p. 3, January 6, 1972.
30. Medicaid: No damn sense, *New York Times*, p. E7, February 4, 1973.
31. U.S. House Subcommittee on Intergovernmental Relations. *Administration of Federal Health Benefit Programs*, part 3, p. 21. U.S. Government Printing Office, Washington, D.C., 1970.
32. Fitch, R. H. Ross Perot: America's first welfare billionaire. *Ramparts* 10(5): 42-51, 1971.
33. Congress approves Social Security bill with Medicare and Medicaid amendments. *Washington Report on Medicine and Health*, October 23, 1972.
34. States struggling with Medicaid crisis. *American Medical News* 14: 1, January 25, 1971.
35. Medicaid: Why the program is mortally ill. *New York Times*, p. E4, October 17, 1971.
36. Proposed Blue Cross rate rise protested by subscribers' unit. *New York Times*, p. 7, January 6, 1971.
37. Katz, D. UAW aide blasts request by Blues for rate hikes. *Detroit Free Press* 140: 1, December 30, 1970.
38. Consumer suits filed against Colorado plans. *The Blue Shield* 9: 3, February 19, 1973.
39. Denenberg, H. Blue Shield debate need for "reform." *American Medical News* 15: 10, October 9, 1972.
40. Denenberg on the rampage. *Medical World News*, pp. 43-50, March 16, 1973.
41. Concessions from a consumer advocate. *Medical World News*, p. 78, October 12, 1973.

84 / Bodenheimer, Cummings, and Harding

42. Survey indicates increased public representation. *The Blue Shield* 8: 4, September 1972.
43. Katz, D. State doctors told to resist Medicaid plan. *Detroit Free Press* 142: 4a, October 5, 1972.
44. Pennsylvania doctors demand ouster of official, talk of boycott. *Washington Post*, p. A2, October 31, 1972.
45. *Materials on Prepaid Health Plans.* Health Policy Advisory Council, San Francisco, 1973.
46. Carnoy, J., et al. Corporate medicine: The Kaiser health plan. *Health/PAC Bulletin*, November 1973.
47. Health Roundup. *Health Security News* 3(1): 4, January 1974.
48. The health bill rises. *Health/PAC Bulletin*, March-April 1974.
49. Health care message from the President of the United States. *Congressional Record* 120: H540, February 6, 1974.
50. Americans who lack insurance coverage. *San Francisco Sunday Examiner and Chronicle*, p. A22, May 6, 1973.
51. Testimony of Dr. Amos Johnson, past president of the American Association of General Practice, before the Senate Antitrust and Monopoly Subcommittee, February 24, 1970.
52. A protest on surgery deaths. *San Francisco Chronicle*, p. 10, December 17, 1971.
53. Unneeded surgeries put at 2 million a year. *Washington Post*, p. 1, July 18, 1972.

CHAPTER 6

The Political Economy
of Medical Care

An Explanation of the Composition, Nature, and Functions of the Present Health Sector of the United States

Vicente Navarro

BY WAY OF INTRODUCTION

In trying to understand the present composition, nature, and functions of the health sector in the United States, one is hampered by a great scarcity of literature, both in the sociological and the medical care fields, that would explain how the shape and form of the health sector—the tree—is determined by the same economic and political forces shaping the political and economic system of the United States—the forest. In fact, health services literature reveals what C. W. Mills (1), Birnbaum (2), and others (3, 4) have found in other areas of social research: a predominance of empiricism, leading to dominance of experts on trees who neither analyze nor question the forest but accept it as given.

Health services research, like most social research, has become more and more compartmentalized, with its practitioners turning into narrower and narrower specialists, superbly trained in their own fields, but with less and less comprehension of the total. And yet, the Hegelian dictum that "the truth is the whole" continues with its undiminished validity. Let me underline that I am not belittling empirical studies, i.e. the analysis of detail. Actually, the reader will see that I borrow heavily from the findings of empirical studies. But, as Baran and Sweezy (5) have indicated, "just as the

This chapter is based on a presentation at the Annual Conference of the New York Academy of Medicine, April 25-26, 1974. A modified version of the article has appeared in the *Bulletin of the New York Academy of Medicine*.

whole is always more than the sum of the parts, so the amassing of small truths about the various parts and aspects of society can never yield the big truths about the social order itself." There is, indeed, a need for explanation of how the parts are related to each other, and it is in meeting this need that our empiricists have fallen short and, for the most part, have remained silent. It is to break this deafening silence that this article has been written. Although admittedly full of assumptions, perceptions, and values, it will try to show that the composition and distribution of health resources is determined by the same forces that determine the distribution of economic and political power in our society. Indeed, I would postulate that the former cannot be understood without an understanding of the latter.

The article is divided into three sections. The first is an analysis of the current social classes and economic structures of the United States, both outside and within the health sector. The second analyzes the different degrees by which social class influences and controls the financing and delivery of care in health institutions, and the third analyzes the effects of class on the organs of the state. It is theorized that these social class influences on the institutions of production, reproduction, and legitimization determine the composition, nature, and functions of the health sector.

THE CLASS STRUCTURE OF THE UNITED STATES, OUTSIDE AND WITHIN THE HEALTH SECTOR

In attempting to explain and understand the composition, functions, and nature of the health sector, one must look outside the health sector and first address a key question in any society, i.e. who owns and who controls the income and wealth of that society?[1] Thus, I have to revive a forgotten paradigm in social analysis in the United States: that of social class structure. In so doing, I am going against the mainstream of our sociological research, which assumes that this category has been transcended by the present reality of the United States, where it is considered that most of our population is middle class. Actually, it is assumed in most of the press and in most of academia that the contemporary United States, and the rest of the western democracies for that matter, are being recast in a mold of middle-class conditions and styles of life.[2] Moreover, this situation is considered to be the result of social fluidity and mobility that is believed to falsify past characterizations of the United States as a class society. This conclusion, however, seems to confuse class consciousness with class interests. Indeed, the social reality that establishes the level of social aspiration of the American population as the consumption pattern of the middle class, and the assumed concomitant absence of class consciousness, do not deny the existence of social classes. In fact, as C. W. Mills (9) pointed out,

> ... the fact that men are not "class conscious" at all times and in all places does not mean that "there are no classes" or that "in America everybody is middle class." The economic and social facts are one thing. Psychological feelings may or may not be associated with them in rationally expected ways. Both are important, and if psychological feelings and political outlooks do not correspond to economic or

[1] Simply stated, income is money coming from different sources, either as wages and salaries, dividends and profits, or as rent. Wealth is the value of people's possessions and property.

[2] An example of a recent newspaper article exhibiting this belief is that by Kumpa (6). The most influential of the large body of sociological literature that negates the existence of classes in the United States is D. Bell (7). For a critique of this literature, see reference 8.

occupational class, we must try to find out why, rather than throw out the economic baby with the psychological bath, and so fail to understand how either fits into the national tub.

Actually, there is not even convincing evidence that class consciousness or awareness do not exist. According to a study conducted in 1964, 56 per cent of all Americans said that they thought of themselves as "working class," some 39 per cent considered themselves "middle class," and 1 per cent said they were "upper class." Only 2 per cent rejected the whole idea of class (10).

An analysis of the social structure of the United States shows that there are indeed social classes in this country. There are a relatively small number of people on the top who own a markedly disproportionate share of personal wealth and whose income is largely derived from ownership. Many of these owners also control the uses to which their assets are put. But, increasingly, this control is vested in people who, although wealthy themselves, do not personally own more than a small part of the assets they control—the managers of that wealth. Both the owners and controllers of wealth constitute what can be defined as the upper class, or for reasons to be defined later, the corporate class, and they command, by virtue of ownership or control or both, the most important sectors of economic life. Actually, according to Lampman (11), the most complete study of the distribution of ownership of wealth ever undertaken in the United States showed that in 1956 the wealthiest 1.6 per cent of the population owned at least 80 per cent of all corporate stocks (the most important type of income-producing wealth) and virtually all state and local government bonds. And, although no subsequent studies have been done on individual ownership of wealth, it seems highly unlikely that this high concentration of economic wealth has changed between 1956 and the present time (12). A similar concentration appears in the distribution of income. Actually, Samuelson (13), using one of his excellent graphic analogies, makes this quite clear in the Eighth Edition of *Economics* when he states that "if we made today an income pyramid out of a child's blocks, with each layer portraying $1,000 of income, the peak would be far higher than the Eiffel Tower, but almost all of us would be within a yard of the ground."

At the other end of the social scale is the working class, composed primarily of industrial or blue-collar workers, the workers of the services sector, and also the agricultural wage earners, although the latter form a steadily decreasing part of the labor force.[3] In 1970 these groups represented 35 per cent, 12 per cent, and 1.8 per cent of the labor force, respectively (15). This working class remains everywhere a distinct and specific social formation "by virtue of a combination of characteristics which affect its members in comparison with the members of other classes" (14, p. 16). It is also primarily from their ranks that the unemployed, the poor, and the subproletariat come.

In between the "polar" classes, there is the middle class, consisting of (1) the professionals, including doctors, lawyers, academicians, etc., whose main denominator is that their work is intellectual as opposed to manual, and whose work usually

---

[3] In my categorization of classes, and the strata within classes, I have very closely followed Chapter 2, "Economic Elites and Dominant Classes," pp. 23-48, in R. Miliband (14). It is recognized that this categorization is far from complete, comprehensive, or even all-inclusive. Still, with all its limitations, it is presented in this article as an entry point to our understanding of the composition of the labor force in the health sector and of the distribution of economic and political power both outside and within the health sector.

requires a professional training; (2) the business middle class, associated with small and medium-sized enterprises, ranging from businessmen employing a few workers to owners of fairly sizeable enterprises of every kind, and who are the owners and controllers of O'Connor's competitive sector (16, pp. 13-15) or of Galbraith's market sector of our economy (17, pp. 55-71); (3) the self-employed shopkeepers, craftsmen, and artisans, a declining sector of the labor force, representing less than 8 per cent of that force; and (4) the office and sales workers (the majority of the white-collar workers), the group that has increased most rapidly within the labor force in the last two decades and that today represents almost a quarter of the labor force of the United States and of most Western European countries (18). In terms of income, in 1970 their median income, at $6,500 per worker, was closer to the blue-collar worker's median income of $6,000, and to the service worker's $4,000, than to the median income of any of the other three middle-class groups, e.g. the median income of the professionals, which was $18,000 (19, 20).

For reasons of brevity, and accepting the simplifications that this categorization implies, I will continue in this paper to refer to groups (1) and (2) as the upper middle class and groups (3) and (4) as the lower middle class. Table 1 shows, in summary form,

Table 1

Occupational and social class distribution in the United States[a]

DISTRIBUTION OF THE LABOR FORCE		SOCIAL CLASS	ESTIMATED ANNUAL MEDIAN INCOME
PERCENTAGE	OCCUPATIONAL GROUP		
1.3%	CORPORATE OWNERS and MANAGERS	CORPORATE CLASS	$ 80-100,000
14%	PROFESSIONALS and TECHNICALS	UPPER MIDDLE CLASS	18,000
6%	BUSINESS MIDDLE CLASS EXECUTIVES		16,000
7%	SELF-EMPLOYED, SHOP-KEEPERS, CRAFTSMEN, and ARTISANS	LOWER MIDDLE CLASS	8,500
23%	CLERICAL and SALES WORKERS		6,500
35%	MANUAL WORKERS	WORKING CLASS	6,000
12%	SERVICE WORKERS		4,000
1.8%	FARM WORKERS		2,600

[a]Sources, references 15, 19, and 20; A. Giddens, *The Class Structure of the Advanced Societies.* Hutchinson University Press, New York, 1973.

the percentage of the population and of the labor force in each occupational category and each social class and gives the annual median income for each category.

The distributions of wealth and income follow these class lines, with the highest possession of both at the top and the lowest possession at the bottom. Moreover, these distribution patterns of wealth and income have remained remarkably constant over time. In the last retrospective study of the distribution of income, published in the 1974 annual *Economic Report of the President* (21), and widely reported in the press, it was found that "the bottom 20 per cent of all families had 5.1 per cent of the nation's income in 1947 and had almost the same amount, 5.4 per cent, in 1972. At the top, there was a similar absence of significant change. The richest 20 per cent had 43.3 per cent of the income in 1947 and 41.4 per cent in 1972" (22).

This class structure in our society is also reflected in the composition of the different elements that participate in the health sector, either as owners, controllers, or producers of services. Indeed, considering just the health sector, and analyzing the owners, controllers, and producers of services in health institutions, we find that members of the upper class and, to a lesser degree, the upper middle class (groups 1 and 2 of the middle class in the previous categorization), predominate in the decision-making bodies of our health institutions, i.e. the boards of trustees of foundations, teaching hospital institutions, medical schools, and hospitals. For the producers and the members of the labor force in the health sector we can see the distribution shown in Figure 1. At the top we find the physicians, who are mainly of upper-middle-class backgrounds and who had in 1970 a median annual net income of $40,000, which places them in the top 5 per cent of our society. I should add that the majority of persons in this group are white and male, besides being upper middle class. They represent 7.3 per cent of the whole labor force in the health sector.

Below, very much below the upper class of the health sector, we find the level called paraprofessional. This could be defined as equivalent to the lower-middle-class category of office worker of the previous categorization (group 4), i.e. nurses, therapists, technologists, and technicians, whose annual median income was approximately $6,000 in 1970. They represent 28.5 per cent of the labor force in the health sector. This group is primarily female and is part of the lower-income group. Nine per cent is black.

Below this group we find the working class per se of the health sector, the auxiliary, ancillary, and service personnel, representing 54.2 per cent of the labor force, who are predominantly women (84.1 per cent) and who include an overrepresentation of blacks (30 per cent). This group's median income was $4,000 in 1970.

If we look at income distribution in the health sector, as we did for society in general, we find a similar structure, although here again, we find a great scarcity of information and a great absence of empirical data. Figure 2, however, shows the trend in the differentials of median income among the different groups of producers in the health sector from 1949 to 1970. Here we can see that there has been a very dramatic increase in the income differential between the top and bottom income groups of the health industry.

The Determinants of Income Differentials

Much has been written about the reasons for these income differentials. According to the orthodox economic paradigm, "every agent of production receives the amount

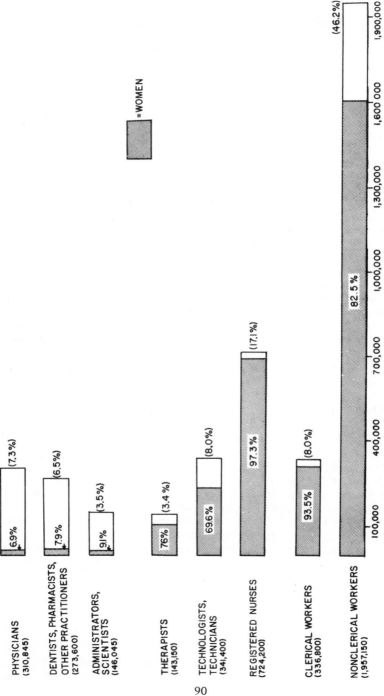

PHYSICIANS
(310,845)
6.9% (7.3%)

DENTISTS, PHARMACISTS,
OTHER PRACTITIONERS
(273,600)
7.9% (6.5%)

ADMINISTRATORS,
SCIENTISTS
(146,045)
9.1% (3.5%)

THERAPISTS
(143,150)
76% (3.4%)

TECHNOLOGISTS,
TECHNICIANS
(341,400)
69.6% (8.0%)

REGISTERED NURSES
(724,200)
97.3% (17.1%)

CLERICAL WORKERS
(336,800)
93.5% (8.0%)

NONCLERICAL WORKERS
(1,957,150)
82.5% (46.2%)

= WOMEN

100,000   400,000   700,000   1,000,000   1,300,000   1,600,000   1,900,000

90

Figure 1. Persons employed in the delivery of health services in the United States, by sex, in 1970. Source for numbers of persons employed in the health services, Health Services and Mental Health Administration, *Health Resources Statistics: Health Manpower and Health Facilities, 1971*, U.S. Government Printing Office, Washington, D.C., 1972. Source for percentage of women physicians, M. Y. Pennell and J. E. Renshaw, Distribution of women physicians, 1970, *Journal of the American Medical Women's Association 27*(4): 197-203, 1972. Source for other categories, U.S. Bureau of the Census, 1970.

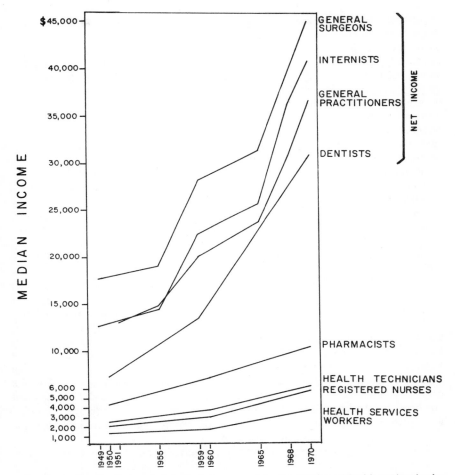

Figure 2. The rise in income of selected personnel in the delivery of health services in the United States, 1949-1970. Source for income of physicians, Continuing Survey of Physicians, Medical Economics Company, Oradell, N. J., 1972. Figures are for self-employed physicians in solo practice, under age 65. Source for income of dentists, Continuing Survey of Dentists, *Journal of the American Dental Association*, various years. Source for income of other wage groups, U.S. Bureau of the Census, *Statistical Abstract of the United States*, U.S. Government Printing Office, Washington, D. C. 1950, 1960, and 1970.

of wealth that agent creates" and "every man receives all that he creates." Thus, workers' incomes depend on their productivity, i.e. "on the amount of capital available, on the one hand, and on workers' skills and education, on the other."[4] According to this interpretation, the conditions for social mobility are (a) increased education, to improve the workers' position in the market for their skills, and (b) equal

[4] All these quotations are from J. B. Clark (23). The marginal productivity of income distribution was first enunciated by Clark in this work. The most important contemporary work in this area is Samuelson (13).

opportunity for each worker in the competitive labor market. The strategy, then, is to increase educational opportunities and to break with the race and sex discrimination which prevents the proper functioning of the market forces. This paradigm is shared, incidentally, by the majority of people in the black and women's liberation movements within and outside the health sector. However, absent in this analysis is the concept of property and class. Actually, one of the widely accepted theoretical works on social inequality in today's United States, Rawls' *A Theory of Justice* (24), does not even mention the value of property as a source of social cleavage. Indeed, following the Weberian interpretation of status, Rawls and most of the exponents of what Barry (25) calls the liberal paradigm maintain that social stratification is multidimensional, depending on a variety of factors such as education, income, occupation, religion, ethnicity, and so on (26).

Empirical evidence, however, seems to question the main assumptions of the liberal paradigm. Regarding the social mobility that is supposed to be the result of the widening of opportunities and of the free flow of labor market forces, and that is supposed to have caused the withering away of the social classes, Westergaard (27) and others have recently shown that although there has been some mobility among the different social groups or strata within each social class, there has been practically no mobility among social classes.

And the primary objective of education, instead of being the transmission of skills to aid upward mobility, seems to have been the perpetuation of social roles within the predefined social classes. Indeed, Bowles and Gintis (28), among others, have indicated how education, labor markets, and industrial structures interact to produce distinctive social strata *within* each class. A similar situation prevails in the health sector, where Simpson (29) and Robson (30) in England, and Kleinbach (31) in the United States have shown how (a) the social class background of the main groups within the health labor force has not changed during the last 25 years, and how (b) education fixes and perpetuates those social backgrounds and replicates social roles. Actually, let me point out here that Flexner himself saw that as a function of medical education when he wrote that a primary aim of medical education was to separate the gentlemen (the upper class) from the quacks (the lower class).

Education, as a perpetuation of social roles, remains the same today as in Flexner's time. Simpson (29, p. 39), for instance, mentions that, within the five-scale grouping of classes in Britain, the offspring of social classes 1 and 2 (equivalent to our upper and upper middle classes, as defined before) predominate in medicine:

> In 1961 more than a third were from class 2, rather less than a third from class 3, and only 3 per cent from classes 4 and 5 together. By 1966, social class 1 was contributing nearly 40 per cent. The proportion of children of classes 1 and 2 in universities generally, derived from the Robbins Report, is about 59 per cent. Individual medical schools vary between 69 and 73 per cent. It is hard to believe that the small number of medical students selected from families of low average income exhausts the potentially good students contained in this large part of the population.

That this situation may even follow a predefined policy is indicated in the following statement from the Royal College of Surgeons (32):

> ... there has always been a nucleus in medical schools of students from cultured homes .... This nucleus has been responsible for the continued high social prestige of the profession as a whole and for the maintenance of medicine as a learned profession.

Medicine would lose immeasurably if the proportion of such students in the future were to be reduced in favour of the precocious children who qualify for subsidies from the Local Authorities and State purely on examination results.

A similar situation occurs in the United States, where Lyden, Geiger, and Peterson (33) reported in 1968 that only 17 per cent of physicians were the children of craftsmen or skilled and unskilled laborers (who represented 57 per cent of the whole labor force), while over 31 per cent of physicians were children of professionals (representing 4.9 per cent of the labor force). Actually, it is quite interesting and, I would add, not surprising, to note that while the underrepresentation of women and blacks among new entrants to the medical schools slowly, but steadily, diminished over the last decade, the underrepresentation of entrants with working-class and lower-middle-class backgrounds remained remarkably constant during the same period (34). Indeed, women, who represent 51 per cent of the U.S. population, made up 6 per cent of all medical students in 1961 and 16 per cent in 1973, while blacks, representing 12 per cent of the overall U.S. population, went during the same time period from 2 to 6 per cent of all medical students. During these years the percentage of medical students who came from families earning the median family income or below, representing approximately one-half of the population, remained at 12 per cent. This percentage, incidentally, has remained the same since 1920.

These accumulated bits of evidence would seem to indicate that there is not an automatic trend toward diminishing class differences or bringing about social class mobility within and outside the health sector of the present United States, and, I would postulate, in that of most Western European societies. As in the past, experience seems to show that, as Harold Laski used to say, "the careful selection of one's own parents," remains among the most important variables explaining one's own power, wealth, income, and opportunities. The importance of this selection, moreover, seems to be particularly vital at the top. As C. W. Mills (35) said, "It is very difficult to climb to the top . . . it is much easier and much safer to be born there."

It would seem, then, that the liberal paradigm does not sufficiently explain the composition of the labor force and its class and income structure. Indeed, I would postulate that a better explanation of that structure would be that the inequalities of income, wealth, and, as we will see in a later section, economic and political power, are functionally related to the way in which the means of production and reproduction of goods, commodities, and services, and the organs of legitimization in the United States, are owned, controlled, influenced, and directed. According to this interpretation, property and control of, and/or influence on, those means of production, reproduction, and legitimization are not just marginal factors in explaining class structure and income differentials, as the liberal paradigm would suggest, but key explanatory ones. Thus, in this alternative explanation, the overall distribution of wealth and income depends on who owns, controls, influences, and directs the means of production, reproduction, and legitimization in the different sectors of the U.S. economy. Overall income differentials among social classes, then, do not have so much to do with the free operation of the labor market forces, but more with the patterns of ownership and control of the main means of income-producing wealth and of the organs of legitimization, i.e. communication, education, and the agencies of the state.[5]

---

[5] The term "state" includes those institutions—the executive, the legislature, the military and police, and the judicial branch—whose interrelationships shape the form of the state system (14).

And according to this alternate explanation, education and other means of socialization are not the means of creating upward mobility among social classes, but actually are means of perpetuating patterns of control and ownership.

In summary, it can be postulated that social classes and income differentials come about because of the different degrees of ownership, control, and influence that different social classes have over the means of production and consumption and over the organs of legitimization, including the media, communications, education, and even the organs of state. Moreover, it can further be postulated that, as I will try to show in the following sections, these class influences determine not only the nature of the economic sectors in the United States today but also of the social sectors, including that of the health services. But, before discussing this, allow me to briefly outline the different sectors of our economy and their class composition, as a necessary prologue to explaining the nature, role, and functions of the health sector.

The Monopolistic, Competitive, and State Sectors of the U.S. Economy

O'Connor (16) and Galbraith (17), among others, have recently defined three different sectors in the United States economy: the planned or monopolistic sector, the market or competitive sector, and the state sector.

The first, the *planned or monopolistic sector,* which roughly employs a third of the labor force, is characterized by being capital- as opposed to labor-intensive, national in contrast to regional or local, and highly monopolistic both in economic concentration and in economic behavior (e.g. in the use of price fixing). Important characteristics of this sector are its requirements for economic stability and planning and a tendency toward vertical integration (e.g. the control of raw materials from the point of extraction to the process of production and distribution) as well as horizontal integration (i.e. the control of different vertical sectors of the industry and the establishment of conglomerates). If we look at the social makeup of this sector, we find (1) the corporation owners (the stockholders) and the controllers (or managers), who Galbraith (17) says together make up the "corporate community" and whom Miliband (14) labels the "large business community," and whom, according to my own definition outlined before, we would call the corporate class; (2) the technocracy or professionals, group 1 of our categorization of the middle class; (3) the blue-collar workers, highly unionized in this sector, who correspond to the industrial working class of my previous categorization; and (4) the white-collar workers, the technical and administrative workers, or lower middle class.

The second sector, the *market or competitive sector,* used to be the largest of the three sectors but today is the smallest and continues to decline. It employs roughly less than one-third of our labor force, with the largest proportion of workers being in services and distribution (16). It is characterized by being labor-intensive, local or regional in scope, with a relatively weak labor force and low unionization. Examples of workers in this sector are people working in restaurants, drug stores, commercial display, etc. The social makeup of this sector consists of (1) the owners and controllers (executives) of small-scale, localized industries and services, group 2 of our own categorization of the upper middle class, (2) small percentages of blue-collar workers and (3) of white-collar workers, and (4) a large sector of service workers, who are primarily auxiliary and ancillary personnel.

The third major sector is the *state sector,* which is made up of two subsectors. The

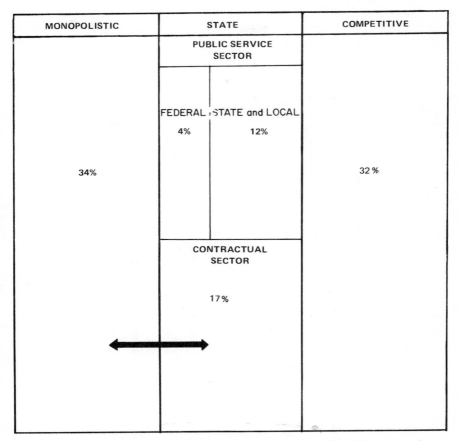

Figure 3. Approximate percentage of labor force in each sector of the U.S. economy. Sources, references 16 and 20.

first subsector produces goods and services under the direction of the state itself, e.g. the public health services, and the second involves production organized by industries under contract from the state. The contracts, e.g. for military equipment and supplies, are mainly with corporations belonging to the monopolistic sector. In terms of social makeup, the first subsector, employing close to 17 per cent of the labor force, has characteristics similar to those of the market system, while the other—the contractual one—also employs 17 per cent of the labor force and is part of the monopolistic sector. Figure 3 summarizes the percentage of the labor force in each sector and Table 2 the main characteristics of the production and labor force in each sector.

Of these three sectors, the most important one for an explanation of the present economic system of the United States and also, according to my postulate, for a partial explanation of the situation in the health field, is the monopolistic sector. Actually, the owners and controllers of that sector, the American corporate class, have a pervasive and constantly felt dominant influence over the patterns of production and

Table 2

Production and labor force characteristics of each sector of the U.S. economy

	MONOPOLISTIC	STATE		COMPETITIVE
	CONTRACTUAL	SERVICE		
CHARACTERISTICS OF PRODUCTION	• PRIMARILY MANUFACTURING • ECONOMIC CONCENTRATION • HIGHLY MONOPOLISTIC • VERTICAL and HORIZONTAL INTEGRATION (CONGLOMERATES) • NATIONAL and INTERNATIONAL	• PRIMARILY SERVICE • ECONOMIC DECONCENTRATION • MONOPOLISTIC • VERTICAL and SECTORIAL • FEDERAL, STATE, LOCAL		• PRIMARILY TRADE and SERVICE • ECONOMIC DECONCENTRATION • COMPETITIVE • VERTICAL and SECTORIAL • REGIONAL and LOCAL
CHARACTERISTICS OF LABOR FORCE	• PREDOMINANTLY MALE • NONWHITES: UNDERREPRESENTED • UNIONIZED • SALARIES: RELATIVELY HIGH	• PREDOMINANTLY FEMALE • NONWHITES: PROPORTIONALLY REPRESENTED • NONUNIONIZED • SALARIES: MEDIUM		• PREDOMINANTLY FEMALE • NONWHITES: OVERREPRESENTED • NONUNIONIZED • SALARIES: LOW

consumption of the United States.[6] Their influence affects the most important means of production and distribution in the United States, as well as the means of value generation, including the media and the educational institutions, and the organs of the state.

I believe that in the health sector, that same class, augmented in this case by the upper middle classes (the professionals and the business middle class of my categorization), maintains a dominant influence on (a) the financial and health delivery institutions, (b) the health teaching institutions, and (c) the organs of the state in the health sector.[7]

THE CONTROL OF THE FINANCIAL AND
HEALTH DELIVERY INSTITUTIONS

The Structure of the Monopolistic Sector and Its Meaning in the Health Sector of the United States

A main characteristic of the economies of the United States and most western nations is the high concentration of economic wealth in the monopolistic sector. Table 3, for instance, shows the extremely high concentration of corporate assets in comparatively few firms. In 1967, at the top a few giant corporations (958, or just 0.06 per cent) held a majority of all assets ($1,070 billion, or 53.2 per cent), while at the bottom, a large number of small corporations (906,458, or 59 per cent of the total) held a very small, almost minuscule portion of corporate assets ($31 billion, or 1.5 per cent).

Table 3

Distribution of corporate assets for all U.S. corporations in 1967[a]

Minimum Assets	Corporations	Assets Owned
$	%	%
0	59.00	1
100,000	29.00	5
500,000	10.00	10
5,000,000	1.94	31
250,000,000	0.06	53
Total	100.00	100

[a]Source, data from U.S. Internal Revenue Service: Statistics of Income, *Corporation Income Tax Returns*. U.S. Government Printing Office, Washington, D. C., 1967.

[6] By dominant or hegemonic influence I mean that influence which is most important in determining "an order in which a certain way of life and thought is dominant, in which one concept of reality is diffused throughout society in all its institutional and private manifestations, informing with its spirit all taste, morality, customs, religious and political principles, and social relations, particularly in their intellectual and moral connotations" (36).

[7] In this article I will limit myself to an analysis of the influence of the corporate classes and upper middle classes on the federal executive and legislative.

This concentration of corporate economic power replicates itself in the several sectors that constitute the United States economy. For example, in the key sector of manufacturing, in 1962 a mere 100 firms (out of a total of 180,000 corporations and 240,000 unincorporated businesses) owned 58 per cent of the net capital assets of all the hundreds of thousands of manufacturing corporations. Another way of expressing this extraordinary degree of concentration is that, as Hunt and Sherman (37, p. 270) point out, "the largest 20 manufacturing firms owned a larger share of the assets than the smallest 419,000 firms combined."[8]

Another sector within the corporate side of the economy is the financial capital sector, which includes the banks, trusts, and insurance companies. Highly concentrated itself (according to the Pattman report (39) the 100 largest banks—out of a total of 13,775 commercial banks—hold 45 per cent of all deposits), this group exerts a dominant influence in the corporate sector, primarily through lending to the corporations. Actually, as a Congressional Committee report (38) indicated recently, accumulated evidence shows that corporations are not self-sufficient in terms of financial capital, but are increasingly dependent on the financial institutions for their capital needs. This dependency leads to influence on corporate policies by the financial capital institutions, through ownership of corporate stocks and the interlocking of directorships in their boards. As Morton Mintz (40) of the *Washington Post* wrote in summarizing the findings of that report, "Most of the nation's largest corporations appear to be dominated or controlled by eight institutions, including six banks." Through their boards, these banks have a close interlocking relationship with insurance companies such as Aetna Life, Prudential, and others. And it may give you an idea of the formidable concentration of power in those finance institutions when I tell you that, again according to that report, the top four banks in the country own 10 per cent of ITT stocks, 12 per cent of Xerox, 22 per cent of Gulf Oil, 10 per cent of International Paper, 12 per cent of Polaroid, and parts of many, many other powerful corporations. The importance of these figures may be shown by the fact that the House Banking and Currency Subcommittee of the U.S. Congress has stated that a 5 per cent ownership of stock in a corporation is sufficient to give the owners of the stock a controlling vote in that corporation (40).

Not surprisingly, the top financial institutions are also important in the health industry, the second largest industry in the country. According to the *National Journal* (41), the flow of health insurance money through private insurance companies in 1973 was $29 billion, slightly less than half of the total insurance—health and other—sold in this country in that year. About $15 billion, or over half of this money, flowed through the commercial insurance companies. Among these companies, we find, again, a high concentration of financial capital, with the ten largest commercial health insurers (Aetna, Travellers, Metropolitan Life, Prudential, CNA, Equitable, Mutual of Omaha, Connecticut General, John Hancock, and Provident) controlling close to 60 per cent of the entire commercial health insurance industry. Most of these top health insurance companies are also the biggest life insurance companies, which are, with the banks, the most important controllers of financial capital in this country. Metropolitan Life and Prudential, for instance, each control $30 billion in assets, making them far larger than General Motors, Standard Oil of New Jersey, and ITT (42). These

---

[8] There are several references showing the concentration of corporate wealth in this country. See the chapter "Monopoly Power: Increasing or Decreasing?" pp. 267-282, in Hunt and Sherman (37) and also reference 38.

financial entities have close links with banking, and through the banks they exercise a powerful influence over the top corporations. An example of this influence is that, out of 28 directors of Metropolitan Life, 23 also sit on the boards of banking institutions, particularly of the Chase Manhattan Bank (42), which owns 10 per cent of the stocks of American Airlines, 8 per cent of those of United Airlines, 15 per cent of the Columbia Broadcasting System, 6 per cent of Mobil Oil, and portions of very many other corporations (40). The importance of this influence, defined by some, such as the Subcommittee on Government Operations of the U.S. Senate, as dominance over the overall economy, is reflected in the present debate on the different proposals for national health insurance, on whether to "open the doors" to the commercials or keep them out of the coming national health insurance scene. It actually speaks highly of the great political influence and power of these financial capital institutions that all the proposals, with the exception of the Kennedy-Griffith proposal whose main constituency was the trade unions of the monopolistic sector, i.e. AFL-CIO and UAW, have left room for, and even encouraged, the involvement of the commercials in the health sector. The Nixon, and now the Ford administration's proposal, for example, would increase the flow of money through the private insurance industry (including commercial health insurance) from $29 to $42 billion, with another $14 billion handled by the private carriers in their role as intermediaries in the publicly financed segment of the proposed plan (41). Actually, it was the power of the commercial insurance companies that determined a change in the Kennedy-Griffith proposal—the only proposal which excluded the insurance companies—to one of acceptance of their role in the new Kennedy-Mills proposal. In fact, as a recent editorial in the *New York Times* (43) indicated, the decision of the Kennedy-Mills proposal "to retain the insurance companies' role was based on recognition of that industry's power to kill any legislation it considers unacceptable. The bill's sponsors thus had to choose between appeasing the insurance industry and obtaining no national health insurance at all."

We can see, then, how the same financial and corporate forces that are dominant in shaping the American economy also increasingly shape the health services sector. The commercial insurance companies, however, although the largest financial power in the premium market in the health sector, are not the only ones. They compete with the power of the providers, expressed in the insurance sector primarily through the Blues—Blue Cross and Blue Shield. The controllers of both the commercials and the Blues, although sharing class interests, have opposite and conflicting corporate interests. Actually, it is likely that the predominance of financial capital in the health sector, and specifically of commercial insurance, could mean the weakening of the providers' control of the health sector, analogous to the way in which the predominance of the monopolistic sector—financial and corporate—has meant the weakening of the market or competitive sector. If this should come about, we would probably see the proletarianization of the providers, with providers being mere employees of the finance corporations—the commerical insurance companies. In this respect, unionization of the medical profession would be a symptom of its proletarianization, so that the present incipient but steady trend toward unionization of the medical profession may be an indication of things to come in the health sector (44).

The Control of the Health Institutions: The Reproductory Ones

In order to understand the patterns of control and/or influence in the health sector, we have to look not only at the patterns of control in the financing of health services, but also at the patterns of control and influence in the health delivery institutions. Indeed, financial capital, the money or energy that moves the system, goes through prefixed institutional channels that are owned, controlled, and/or influenced by classes and groups which are similar to, although not identical with, those who have dominant influence through financing. We can group the institutions into (1) those that have to do with the reproduction and legitimization of the patterns of control and influence, e.g. the teaching institutions, and (2) those that deliver the services themselves. Indeed, following this categorization, we could speak of reproductive versus distributive institutions.

The former, in which I would include the foundations (e.g. the Johnson, Rockefeller, and Carnegie Foundations) besides the teaching medical institutions, are controlled by the financial and corporate communities and by the professionals, i.e. the corporate class and the upper middle class of my initial categorization. As Professor MacIver (45) writes, "in the non-governmental (teaching) institutions, the typical board member is associated with large-scale business, a banker, manufacturer, business executive, or prominent lawyer," to which, in the health sector, we could add a prominent physician. For instance, one study (46) showed that of the 734 trustees of 30 leading universities half were recognized members of the professions, and half were proprietors, managers, and bankers. Incidentally, let me add that it is quite misleading to assume that the class and corporate role of such board members is a passive one or that their function is the one of rubber stamping what the administrators and medical faculty decide. In fact, their assumed passivity is one of delegated control. Actually, it was none other than Flexner (47) who, in a not very frequently quoted part of one of his reports, said that "the influence of the board of trustees ... determines in the social and economic realms an atmosphere of timidity which is not without effect on critical appointments and promotions." Indeed, concerning the highest decisions, theirs is the first and final voice. And their first role, as Galbraith (48) has indicated, is to ensure that "the aims of higher education, of course, are to be attuned to the needs of the industrial (corporate) system" which is usually also referred to as the "private enterprise system." In 1961, Dr. Pusey (49), the then President of Harvard, made this quite explicit when he said in a remarkable speech that "the end of all academic departments ... is completely directed towards making the *private enterprise system* continue to work effectively and beneficially in a very difficult world." This clearly ideological statement, from a supposedly unideological academic leader of a presumably unideological establishment, is meritorious for its clarity, conciseness, and straight-forwardness. In fact, this commitment, which is far more typical than atypical of our academic institutions and foundations, cannot be disassociated from the nature of the predominant membership of the corporate and business leaders in the boards of trustees of academia and foundations. (For an updated analysis of the backgrounds, roles, and educational attitudes of university trustees, see reference 50.) The function and purpose of this dominant influence in the boards of trustees is to perpetuate the sets of values that will optimize their collective benefits as class and as corporate interests.

Allow me to clarify here that I do not believe that there is monopoly control in the value-generating system. However, I do think that the system of influence and control in that system is highly skewed in favor of the corporate and financial value system. And this dominant influence is felt not only in universities, foundations, and institutions of higher learning, but also in most of the value-generating systems, from the media to all other instruments of communication (51). As Miliband (14, p. 238) says, all these value-generating systems do contribute to the

> ... fostering of a climate of conformity, not by the total suppression of dissent, but by the presentation of views which fall outside the consensus as curious heresies, or, even more effectively, by treating them as irrelevant eccentricities, which serious and reasonable people may dismiss as of no consequence. This is very functional [for the system].

Actually, another indication of this dominance of corporate values can be seen in the present debate in academia on national health insurance. In spite of the "hot" debate as to what type and nature of national health insurance "Americans may choose," and in spite of the critical nature of comments about our health sector made by considerable sectors of academia and even the mass media, not one of the proposals and not one report in the media questions the sanctity of the private sector, nor its pattern of control of our health institutions. And a whole series of alternatives that would question the present pattern, such as different types of national health services as opposed to just national health insurance, are not even thought of, or are quickly dismissed as being "un-American." The sanctity of "private enterprise values," however, has more to do with the pattern of control of the value-generating system by the financial and corporate interests than with the genetic-biological structure of the American population. As Marcuse (52) has indicated, the success of the system is to make unthinkable the possibility of its alternatives.

The Control of the Health Distribution Institutions

The voluntary community hospitals are the largest component of the health distribution institutions. Analyzing the boards of trustees of these hospitals, one sees less predominance of the representatives of financial and corporate capital, and more of the upper middle class, and primarily of groups 1 and 2 defined before, i.e. the professionals—especially physicians—and representatives of the business middle class. Even here, the other strata and classes, the working class and lower middle class, which constitute the majority of the U.S. population, are not represented. Not one trade union leader (even a token one), for instance, sits on any board in the hospitals in the region of Baltimore (53). And, of course, even less represented on hospital boards are the unorganized workers. Figure 4 presents a summary of the percentage class distribution of the U.S. labor force, and how the classes are represented on the boards of the reproductive and distributive health institutions.

The False Dichotomy of Providers Versus Consumers

Out of the previous analysis it should be clear that I disagree with most of my colleagues who perceive the present basic dialectical conflict in the health sector of the United States—both in the financing and in the delivery of health services—to be between the consumers and the providers. To me this is a simplification that obfuscates the nature of the distribution of economic and political power in the United States today both inside as well as outside the health sector. Although I would agree that the present delivery system seems to be controlled primarily by the

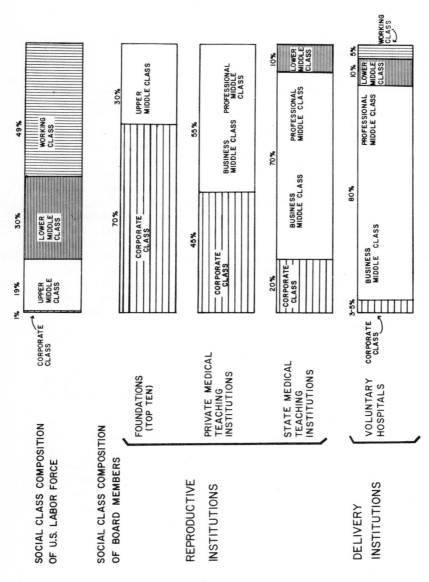

Figure 4. Estimated social class composition of the U.S. labor force and of the boards of trustees of reproductive and delivery institutions in the health sector. Sources, reference 50: V. Navarro, The control of the health institutions, Department of Health Care Organization, Johns Hopkins University, Baltimore (in process); and J. Pfeffer, Size, composition, and functions of hospital boards of directors: A study of organization-environment linkage. *Administrative Science Quarterly* 18(3): 349-364, 1973.

providers and their different components, either the "patricians" or professionals of academia-based medicine, the practitioners or the American Medical Association (AMA), and the hospital organizations or the American Hospital Association (AHA), I would disagree with the proposition that there is an inherent control given to them by their "unique" knowledge or that the situation cannot be changed. Actually, the power of the medical profession is delegated power. As Freidson (54) has indicated, "A profession attains and maintains its position by virtue of the protection and patronage of some elite segment of society which has been persuaded that there is some special value in its work." But as Frankenberg (55) has pointed out, this section or segment of the population is not so much an economic elite as a class, i.e. the corporate class described before. Remember, incidentally, that the Flexner Report and the first scientific medical schools were funded and subsidized by the enlightened establishment of the 1900s, i.e. the Rockefeller and Carnegie Foundations, the intellectual voices of the financial and corporate class of the early 1900s (56).

The great influence of the providers over the health institutions, which amounts to control of the health sector, is based on power delegated from other groups and classes, primarily the corporate class and the upper middle class, to which the providers belong. Their specific interests may actually be in conflict with the power of other groups or strata within the upper middle class and with the greater power of the corporate class. Indeed, as I have indicated elsewhere (57), the corporate powers of England and Sweden not only tolerated, but even supported, the nationalization of the health sector when the corporate interests required it, formalizing a dependency of the medical profession on those corporate and state interests.

To define the main dialectical conflict in the health sector as one of providers versus consumers assumes that (a) providers have the final and most powerful control of decision making in the health sector, and (b) consumers have a uniformity of interests, transcending class and other interests. Control of the health institutions, however, is primarily class control by the classes and groups described before, and only secondarily control by the professions. The dialectical conflicts that exist are not, then, between the providers and the consumers; but instead there is conflict (a) between the corporate class and the providers over the financing of the health sector, and (b) between the majority of the U.S. population, who belong to the working and lower middle classes, and the controllers of the health delivery system—the corporate class and the upper middle class, including the professionals.

THE CORPORATE SYSTEM AND THE STATE

Having described, however briefly, the patterns of influence in both the financing and the delivery systems of the health sector, let me address myself to the final question of our analysis, that of who has dominant influence over the state. Let me add right away that this is far from being a simple question.

Before I attempt to answer the question of who has dominant influence over the state, let me describe what I consider to be erroneous answers. One of these is that government is run by business. As one of the proponents of this theory says, "Government and Congress are run by big business" (58). And actually, this idea is similar to Marx's statement in the *Communist Manifesto* (59) that "the state is the executive committee of the bourgeoisie." It is quite interesting, incidentally, that this view seems to have been held even by past presidents of the United States. Indeed, none other than President Woodrow Wilson said that "the masters of the government of the United States are the combined capitalists and manufacturers of the United States" (quoted in 37, p. 284). However, I find such statements too much of a simplification. But I find equally simplistic the idea, quite prevalent among our scholars, that the state organs are "above" business, or that business is even actually anti-government. I believe this explanation to be unhistorical and unempirical. Actually, in the executive branch of government,

> Businessmen were in fact the largest single occupational group in cabinets from 1889 to 1949; of the total number of cabinet members between these dates, more than 60 per cent were businessmen of one sort or another. Nor certainly was the business membership of American cabinets less marked in the Eisenhower years from 1953 to 1961. As for members of British cabinets between 1886 and 1950, close to one-third were businessmen, including three prime ministers—Bonar Law, Baldwin and Chamberlain. Nor again have businessmen been at all badly represented in the Conservative cabinets which held office between 1951 and 1964 (14, pp. 56-57).

In respect to the legislative branch, in 1970, as Hunt and Sherman (37, p. 288) point out:

> A total of 102 congressmen held stock or well-paying executive positions in banks or other financial institutions; 81 received regular income from law firms that generally represented big businesses. Sixty-three got their income from stock in the top defense contractors; 45, in the giant (federally regulated) oil and gas industries; 22, in radio and television companies; 11, in commercial airlines; and 9, in railroads. Ninety-eight congressmen were involved in numerous capital-gains transactions; each of them netted a profit of over $5,000 (and some as high as $35,000).

It is, therefore, difficult to conclude from these figures that businessmen are anti-government. Let me add that these businessmen in the corridors of power may not necessarily think of themselves as business representatives holding state power. But, it is highly unlikely, as Miliband says, that their vision of national interest runs against the interests of the business community. Indeed, values and beliefs do not change when the call of government takes place. The appointment of businessmen to positions of power has also been the practice in the federal health establishment. For instance, out of the last twelve Secretaries of Health, nine have had business backgrounds.

On the other hand, in the dichotomy between business and labor, labor leaders have been a small, very small minority indeed in the key positions of either the executive or legislative branch. Let me add, though, that this situation is far from unique to the United States. In Sweden, painted as a socialist heaven by some, and as a hell by others, the number of workers' sons and daughters among the top Swedish politico-bureaucratic echelons was less than 9 per cent in 1961 (60).

This heavy involvement of businessmen in government, then, makes one begin to question the widely held belief that businessmen are against government. But, on the other hand, this involvement in, and heavy influence on, the state, should not lead to the opposite conclusion that businessmen are the government—or at least not in the way that the land-owning aristocracy was the government in the 18th century. Indeed, sharing the power of government with big business are other groups who represent different interests. In the executive branch of the federal health establishment, for example, powerful groups with whom the businessmen share power are the professionals of academic medicine—the patricians—and, to a lesser degree, the practitioners.

These two groups, while they are not the top decision makers (who are usually businessmen), do control the next-to-top echelons of policy in the executive of the federal health establishment, e.g. they are the Assistant Secretaries of health and below. The medical practitioners, who control the AMA, incidentally, tend to be more influential on the legislative branch of the federal government than on the executive. An example, among many others, showing the differing degrees of influence the AMA has over the two branches of government was the recent decision of Congress to follow the AMA's wishes and exclude the health sector from cost controls despite the very strong opposition to this exclusion from the executive branch. Still another example is that the AMA proposal for national health insurance is the one proposal with most sponsors in the Congress. And this selective attention by some members of the Congress is not without rewards. Actually, the Common Cause list of federal legislators who received AMA contributions during the last national election in 1972 (61) reads like a "Who's Who" of the health sector in the U.S. Congress.

There is indeed a diversity of interests in the health sector. Yet within this diversity that determines the plurality of sources of power in the federal establishment, there is a uniformity that unites these groups and sets them apart from other groups who do not share the basic characteristics, i.e. their social origin, education, and class situation. As Professor Matthews (62) notes:

> Those American political decision-makers for whom this information is available are, with very few exceptions, sons of professional men, proprietors and officials, and farmers. A very small minority are sons of wage-earners, low salaried workers, farm laborers or tenants ... the narrow base from which political decision-makers appear to be recruited is clear.

In fact, the large majority of the governing classes belong, by social origin and by previous occupation, to our corporate and upper middle classes, as defined before.

Let me underline, once again, that I am not implying that the corporate class and the upper middle class, which predominate in, and dominate, the corridors of power, act and behave uniformly on the political scene. Indeed, they represent a plurality of interests that determines what is usually referred to as the political pluralism of our society. This plurality is reflected in the different programs put forward by the main political parties. In that respect, it is far from my intention to imply that all proposals for national health insurance, for example, are the same, or that they represent the same groups. Differences *do* exist. Yet the nature of this political pluralism means that the benefits of the system are consistently skewed in favor of those classes mentioned before. As an American observer (63) has indicated, "The flaw in the pluralistic heaven is that the heavenly chorus sings with a very special accent ... the system is askew, loaded, and unbalanced in favor of a fraction of a minority." Moreover, the political debate which reflects that pluralism takes place within a common understanding and acceptance of certain basic premises and assumptions, which consistently benefit some classes more than others.

Let me add that this situation is not so much because of personalities, but because of the inner logic of the system, i.e. it is a syndrome of the distribution of economic and political power within our system. It is because of this inner logic that, when there is government intervention, the possible benefits of that intervention are not randomly distributed, but are largely very predictable. And the answer to the question of *cui bono*? to whom the goods? is predictably easy. Let me give you an example—that of the fiscal policies in general and of taxation in particular. Titmuss (64) in Britain and Kolko (65) in this country have shown that the two countries' systems of taxation have not weakened the income inequalities in either country but have actually accentuated them. A similar example in the health sector is the system of funding of most of the national health insurance proposals, which for the most part share the common denominator of being regressive (66).

With this introduction, let me describe, as I perceive them, the roles of state intervention as they relate to the health sector. And I postulate that these roles are (a) the legitimization and defense of the private enterprise system, and (b) the strengthening of that system. These categories are somewhat artificial, and thus their separation is one of convenience more than of necessity.

The Legitimization and Defense of the System

According to Weber, the first role of any state is to assure the survival of the economic system. Thus, the main role of the state is the legitimization of the economic and political relationship via the different mechanisms at the state's disposal. These mechanisms range from the exclusive use of force, i.e. the armed forces and police, to the creation of social services, including the development of health services, with very many mechanisms of intervention between these alternatives. Actually, it was none other than Bismarck, the midwife of the welfare state, who first used the social insurance mechanism as a way of coopting the threatening forces to the capitalist system of that time (67). Social security legislation was passed in England and other countries for similar reasons. Let me quote Sigerist (68), that great Hopkins medical historian, in this respect:

> Social-security legislation came in waves and followed a certain pattern. Increased industrialization created the need; strong political parties representing the interests of the workers seemed a potential threat to the existing order, or at least to the traditional system of production, and an acute scare such as that created by the French Commune stirred Conservatives into action and social-security legislation was enacted. In England at the beginning of our century the second industrial revolution was very strongly felt. The Labor Party entered parliament and from a two-party country England developed into a three-party country. The Russian revolution of 1905 was suppressed to be sure, but seemed a dress rehearsal for other revolutions to follow. Social legislation was enacted not by the Socialists but by Lloyd George and Churchill. A third wave followed World War I when again the industries of every warfaring country were greatly expanded, when, as a result of the war, the Socialist parties grew stronger everywhere, and the Russian revolution of 1917 created a red scare from which many countries are still suffering. Again social-security legislation was enacted in a number of countries.

Nor are we strangers to this mechanism in this country. Piven and Cloward (69) have shown, for example, how welfare rolls are—and always have been—raised to reduce unrest among the poor. It was the function of welfare programs to integrate those sectors of the population who have felt increasingly alienated from the political system and to give them the feeling of being a part of the system in which those programs were introduced. As Moynihan has indicated for the anti-poverty programs of the sixties, "They were intended to do no more than ensure that persons excluded from the political process in the South and elsewhere could nevertheless *participate* in the benefits of the community action programs. . . ." (quoted in 69, p. 268).

In that respect, the lateness of the United States to come to the welfare state stage may be due to the lack of pressure, primarily on the corporate class, from any force that could obtain a concession from that class and achieve what the European Left has achieved for its constituents. The potential for threat does exist, however, and the perception of that potential is explicitly manifested in a continuous call for "law and order," and in expressed concern for the disintegration of the system. Indeed, the percentage of the American people who have expressed alienation from, and disillusionment with, their present system of government has achieved a record high in the history of the United States. A Harris Survey of public attitudes prepared for a U.S. Congressional Committee in 1973 (70) concludes that,

> The most striking verdict rendered [in the survey] by the American people—and disputed by their leaders—is a negative one. A majority of Americans display a degree of alienation and discontent [with government] .... [Those] citizens who thought something was "deeply wrong" with their country had become a national majority .... And for the first time in the ten years of opinion sampling by the Harris Survey, the growing trend of public opinion toward disenchantment with government swept more than half of all Americans with it.

A possible response by government to that popular alienation could be the establishment of measures such as income maintenance or national health insurance, aimed at integrating that alienated population into the political system. As the daily press has indicated, the increased attention of Presidents Nixon and Ford to the national health insurance issue on the political scene, and the broadening of benefits, could easily be related to their concern with the alienation of the population from them personally and from the political system in general (71).

The Strengthening of the Private Enterprise System

In creating a welfare state, however, the inner logic of the system, which is a product of the pattern of economic and political power as explained before, determines that the distribution of benefits brought about through that state intervention is likely to benefit some groups more than others. Actually, it is because I believe the system functions in this way that I am skeptical—as are others—that national health insurance will solve what is usually referred to as the "health crisis" in this country. As Bodenheimer rightly points out, it is far from clear whose crisis national health insurance is supposed to solve—that of the financial interests of the insurance industry and of the providers themselves or that of the availability and accessibility needs of the majority of the population. Not surprisingly, after making a comprehensive analysis of the flow of funds in the health sector, Bodenheimer (66) postulates that,

> Just as federal defense appropriations subsidize the military-industrial complex, national health insurance will subsidize the medical-industrial complex.

Let me finish now by underlining, once again, that state intervention is not uniform, since it depends on the interests of the dominant group in the area in dispute. This is shown by the fact that each one of the different power groups in the health sector has put forward its own proposal aimed at optimizing its own interests. Thus, each proposal has a rationale and ideology behind it which respond to the specific economic interests of its proponents. And, again, reflecting the power of the insurance industry, all proposals, except one, have allowed, and even encouraged, the involvement of insurance in the health sector, with state subsidization of the private insurance industry. As Fein (72) has indicated, in commenting on the Administration proposal, it is part and parcel of that proposal's strategy to strengthen the private market in health sector economic affairs. The passing of this proposal, as well as the majority of the others, would strengthen the contractual segment of the state sector that I discussed in a previous section. Indeed, as you may recall, following the categories outlined by O'Connor and Galbraith, I divided the state sector into two subsectors: the contractual part, in which the state contracts with and subsidizes the private sector, primarily the monopolistic or planned sector (such as in the case of the defense industry), and the part that is owned and operated by the public sector per se, with services that are owned and run by the state, such as the public health services.

The first subsector, or contractual one, will be strengthened with the passing of the suggested national health insurance, and would further expand what O'Connor calls the social-industrial complex. The rationale for that involvement, as *Fortune* magazine says, is that,

> Implicit in the governmental appeals for help at all levels is an acknowledgement that large corporations are the major repository of some rather special capabilities that are now required. Business executives are increasingly identified as the most likely organizers of community-action programs, like the Urban Coalition and its local counterparts. Corporate managers often have the special close-quarters knowledge that enables them to visualize opportunities for getting at particular urban problems—e.g., the insurance companies' plans for investments in the slums. Finally, the new "systems engineering" capabilities of many corporations have opened up some large possibilities for dealing with just about any complex social problem (quoted in 16, pp. 55-56).

Medicare and Medicaid have already begun the expansion of the contractual subsector, and the rate of this expansion has established a record for the rate of growth of financial capital in this country. Indeed, from 1970 to 1973 the profits of the private health insurance industry increased by 120 per cent, establishing an all-time record (73, 74).

Another objective of all the national health insurance proposals is to socialize the increasing costs of health insurance, and to stop the increased drain of funds that health costs represent for both capital and labor. In 1966, for example, contributions to health insurance plans exceeded $8 billion or about 40 per cent of total fringe benefit costs (16, p. 142).

The other subsector of the state sector, the public sector (city hospitals, public health service hospitals, and others), will have the responsibility of taking care of the load that is considered unprofitable or less profitable by the private sector. As Roemer and Mera (75) have concisely shown, the patient population of our city hospitals consists for the most part of patients unwanted by the private sector. Thus, in the health sector, there occurs what happens in other sectors. It is the perceived function of the state to strengthen the private sector, through contracts and subsidies, and by taking care of the unwanted responsibilities of the private sector.

In summary, then, the defined patterns of dominance within the organs of the state explain and ensure that state intervention is aimed at (a) legitimizing those patterns of dominance, and (b) strengthening the private sector, and, of course, the groups that have dominance within it. And it is within this context of the functions and goals of state intervention that the debate regarding the different health insurance proposals must be understood. Thus, the arguments of the proponents of the various alternatives are designed to convince the average citizen that the proposed insurance will improve his or her life, and at the same time, to prove that the system is basically responsive to his or her needs. Yet, by the very nature of class dominance within the state, this intervention will predictably benefit some social classes, some economic groups, and some interest groups more than others.

Indeed, that the proposals are more likely to benefit certain social classes more than others can be seen by the proposed system of funding in the majority of national health insurance proposals, based for the most part on either payroll taxes, social security taxes, and/or premiums, or a combination of these, all of them systems of funding that are highly regressive (66). Also, the likely benefit of these proposals to primarily the dominant economic groups in our society is clear in that the majority of proposals rely on the insurance industry to administer the national insurance scheme, thereby guaranteeing not only the continuation of but also a dramatic increase in the flow of money through that industry. The awareness of this possibility by the insurance industry undoubtedly explains the $9 million campaign that the health and life insurance industry budgeted for 1974 and 1975 to "educate" our citizenry, through TV and other media, on the "merits" of having the insurance industry "involved in and responsible for" the administration of the proposed national health insurance schemes (76).

Also, the provider interest groups will likely benefit to a large extent from whatever form of proposal may pass, sometimes sharing those benefits with the insurance industry, and sometimes competing with it for those benefits.

Thus, it is basically the patterns of dominance that condition the possibilities for change and the definitions of what is possible. Within these definitions and within these possibilities for change, it is unlikely, for example, that the funding of whatever insurance that may pass will be progressive, i.e. designed to ensure that the larger burden of the funding will fall on the strongest rather than the weakest shoulders. Also, within the defined boundaries of what is possible and what is not, it is highly improbable, whatever system of control and regulation may evolve, that the patterns of governance of our health institutions will change profoundly and become more responsive and accountable to the majority of those who either work in or are being served by those institutions. And, meanwhile, as all the "political drama and political heat" continue, the life of the average citizen is likely to remain the same. He is likely to repeat the old adage that "the more things change, the more they remain the same."

CONCLUSION

In summary, then, I have tried to show how the same economic and political forces that determine the class structure of the United States also determine the nature and functions of the U.S. health sector. Indeed, the composition, nature, and functions of the latter are the result of the degree of ownership, control, and influence that primarily the corporate and the upper middle classes have on the means of production, reproduction, and legitimization of U.S. society. This interpretation runs contrary to the most prevalent interpretation, which assumes that the "shape and form" of the health sector is a result of American values that prevail in all areas and spheres of American life. But this explanation assumes that values are the cause, and not, as I postulate, a symptom of the distribution of economic and political power in the United States. In fact, that explanation avoids the question of which groups and classes have a dominant influence on the value-generating system and maintain, perpetuate, and legitimize it. According to my interpretation, they are the very same groups and classes that have a dominant influence over the systems of production, reproduction, and legitimization in other areas of the economy, including the organs of the state.

Let me underline, once again, that I do not believe these groups to be uniform, nor their dominant influence to be equivalent to control. Actually, I find this distinction between dominant influence and control a key one that has a number of implications, primarily in the area of strategies for stimulating change. Indeed, there is a plurality of interests among groups and among classes that explains and determines the political pluralism apparent today in the United States. Competition does exist. And a strategist for change has to be aware of and sensitive to the diversity of interests reflected in political debate (57). However, the competition that supports this pluralism is consistently and unavoidably unequal, skewed, and biased in favor of the dominant groups and classes. To quote the excellent description Miliband (14, pp. 164-165) has made of this situation:

> There is competition, and defeats for powerful capitalist interests as well as victories. After all, David did overcome Goliath. But the point of the story is that David was smaller than Goliath and that the odds were heavily against him.

The degree of skewedness in the distribution of economic and political power, both outside and within the health sector, is, as I have tried to show in this presentation, very dramatic indeed. And at a time when much time and energy are spent in academia in debating what might be the most perfect model for the health sector, it might have a salutary effect to underline that more important than the shape of the final product is the issue of who dominates the process. Thus, a primary intent of this presentation has been to show that the presently debated questions of what services to provide, and for whom, will actually be determined by whoever is dominant in the process of defining those questions and of formulating those answers.

Indeed, I have attempted in this paper to put the tree—our health sector—within the setting of the forest—the economic and political structure of our nation. I am aware that I may have left very many areas loosely sketched or not defined at all, but I suppose there are risks in daring to face the totality. And needless to say, I am aware that this analysis is, according to present Parsonian standards of orthodoxy, an "unorthodox" one. But it may in the long term serve as one more effort to question that orthodoxy. Meanwhile, in the short run, I hope it will at least stimulate students of health services to look wider and deeper than just at their own health sector.

Acknowledgments—I want to express my great appreciation to Christopher George for editing this paper, to Janet Archer for preparing the figures and tables, and to Loetta Wallace for assisting and typing the manuscript.

REFERENCES

1. Mills, C. W. *The Sociological Imagination*. Grove Press, New York, 1959.
2. Birnbaum, N. *Toward a Critical Sociology*. Oxford University Press, New York, 1971.
3. Dreitzel, H. P. *On the Social Basis of Politics*. Macmillan Company, New York, 1969.
4. Coulson, M. A., and Riddell, C. *Approaching Sociology: A Critical Introduction*. Routledge and Kegan Paul, London, 1973.
5. Baran, P., and Sweezy, P. *Monopoly Capital*, pp. 2-3. Monthly Review Press, New York, 1968.
6. Kumpa, P. J. Hail to the middle class! *Baltimore Sun* pp. K1 and K3, March 10, 1974.
7. Bell, D. *End of Ideology: On the Exhaustion of Political Ideas in the Fifties*. Free Press, New York, 1960.
8. Parker, R. *The Myth of the Middle Class: Notes on Affluence and Equality*. Liveright, New York, 1972.
9. Horowitz, I. L., editor. *Power, Politics and People: The Collected Essays of C. Wright Mills*, p. 317. Oxford University Press, New York, 1962. (Quoted in R. Miliband, *The State in Capitalist Society: An Analysis of the Western System of Power*, p. 20. Weidenfeld and Nicolson, London, 1969.)

10. Irish, M., and Prothro, J. *The Politics of American Democracy,* p. 38. Prentice-Hall, Englewood Cliffs, N.J., 1965. (Quoted in E. K. Hunt and H. J. Sherman, *Economics: An Introduction to Traditional and Radical Views,* p. 284. Harper and Row, New York, 1972.)
11. Lampman, R. J. *The Share of Top Wealth-Holders in National Wealth, 1922-1956.* Princeton University Press, Princeton, N. J., 1956. (Quoted in E. K. Hunt and H. J. Sherman, *Economics: An Introduction to Traditional and Radical Views,* p. 390. Harper and Row, New York, 1972.)
12. Upton, L., and Lyons, N. *Basic Facts: Distribution of Personal Income and Wealth in the United States.* Cambridge Institute, Cambridge, Mass., 1972.
13. Samuelson, P. *Economics,* Ed. 8, p. 110. McGraw-Hill Book Company, New York, 1972.
14. Miliband, R. *The State in Capitalist Society: An Analysis of the Western System of Power.* Weidenfeld and Nicolson, London, 1969.
15. United States Bureau of the Census. *Statistical Abstract of the United States: 1970,* p. 225. U.S. Government Printing Office, Washington, D. C., 1970.
16. O'Connor, J. *The Fiscal Crisis of the State.* St. Martin's Press, New York, 1973.
17. Galbraith, J. K. *Economics and the Public Purpose.* Houghton-Mifflin Company, Boston, 1973.
18. Dahrendorf, R. Recent changes in the class structure of European societies. *Daedalus* Winter 1964. (Cited in R. Miliband, *The State in Capitalist Society: An Analysis of the Western System of Power.* Weidenfeld and Nicolson, London, 1969.)
19. *Current Population Reports, Consumer Income: Growth Rates in 1939 to 1968 for Persons by Occupation and Industry Groups for the United States.* Series P-60, No. 69, Table A-3, p. 82. U.S. Government Printing Office, Washington, D. C., 1970.
20. Bonnell, V., and Reich, M. *Workers and the American Economy: Data on the Labor Force.* New England Free Press, Boston, 1973.
21. United States Congress. *Economic Report of the President, 1974.* U.S. Government Printing Office, Washington, D. C., 1974.
22. Shanahan, E. Income distribution found unchanged. *New York Times* p. 10, February 2, 1974.
23. Clark, J. B. *The Distribution of Wealth.* Macmillan Company, New York, 1924. (Quoted in B. Silverman and M. Yanowitch, Radical and liberal perspectives on the working class. *Social Policy* 4(4): 40-50, 1974.)
24. Rawls, J. *A Theory of Justice.* Harvard University Press, Cambridge, Mass., 1971.
25. Barry, B. *The Liberal Theory of Justice: A Critical Examination of the Principal Doctrines in "A Theory of Justice" by John Rawls.* Clarendon Press, Oxford, 1972.
26. Silverman, B., and Yanowitch, M. Radical and liberal perspectives on the working class. *Social Policy* 4(4): 40-50, 1974.
27. Westergaard, J. H. Sociology: The myth of classlessness. In *Ideology in Social Science,* edited by R. Blackburn, pp. 119-163. Fontana, New York, 1972.
28. Bowles, S., and Gintis, H. IQ in the U.S. class structure. *Social Policy* 3(4 and 5): 65-96, 1973.
29. Simpson, M. A. *Medical Education: A Critical Approach.* Butterworths, London, 1972.
30. Robson, J. The NHS Company, Inc.? The social consequence of the professional dominance in the National Health Service. *Int. J. Health Serv.* 3(3): 413-426, 1973.
31. Kleinbach, G. Social structure and the education of health personnel. *Int. J. Health Serv.* 4(2): 297-317, 1974.
32. *Evidence of the Royal College of Surgeons to the Royal Commission on Doctors and Dentists Remuneration.* Her Majesty's Stationery Office, London, 1958. (Quoted in J. Robson, The NHS Company, Inc.? The social consequence of the professional dominance in the National Health Service. *Int. J. Health Serv.* 3(3): 413-426, 1973.)
33. Lyden, F. J., Geiger, H. J., and Peterson, O. *The Training of Good Physicians.* Harvard University Press, Cambridge, Mass., 1968. (Cited in M. A. Simpson, *Medical Education: A Critical Approach,* p. 35. Butterworths, London, 1972.)
34. Kleinbach, G. *Social Class and Medical Education.* Department of Education, Harvard University, Cambridge, Mass., 1974.
35. Mills, C. W. *The Power Elite,* p. 39. Oxford University Press, New York, 1956.
36. Williams, G. A. Gramsci's concept of egemonia. *Journal of the History of Ideas* 21(4): 587, 1960.
37. Hunt, E. K., and Sherman, H. J. *Economics: An Introduction to Traditional and Radical Views.* Harper and Row, New York, 1972.
38. Committee on Government Operations of the United States Senate. *Disclosure of Corporate Ownership.* U.S. Government Printing Office, Washington, D. C., 1973.
39. Pattman Committee Staff Report for the Domestic Finance Subcommittee of the House Committee on Banking and Currency. *Commercial Banks and Their Trust Activities; Emerging Influence on the American Economy.* U.S. Government Printing Office, Washington, D. C., 1968.
40. Mintz, M. Eight institutions control most of top firms. *Washington Post* pp. A1 and A16, January 6, 1974.
41. Iglehart, J. K. National insurance plan tops ways and means agenda. *National Journal* 6(11): 387, 1974.

42. Bodenheimer, T., Cummings, S., and Harding, E. Capitalizing on illness: The health insurance industry. *Int. J. Health Serv.* 4(4): 569-584, 1974.
43. Health plan progress. Editorial. *New York Times* p. E16, April 7, 1974.
44. Kelman, S. Toward the political economy of medical care. *Inquiry* 8(3): 30-38, 1971.
45. MacIver, R. M. *Academic Freedom in Our Time,* p. 78. Gordian Press, New York, 1967. (Cited in R. Miliband, *The State in Capitalist Society: An Analysis of the Western System of Power,* p. 251. Weidenfeld and Nicolson, London, 1969.)
46. Beck, H. P. *Men Who Control Our Universities,* p. 51. King's Crown Press, London, 1947.
47. Flexner, A. *Universities: American, English, German,* p. 180. Oxford University Press, New York, 1930.
48. Galbraith, J. K. *The New Industrial State,* p. 370. Houghton-Mifflin Company, Boston, 1967.
49. Pusey, N. M. *Age of the Scholar: Observations on Education in a Troubled Decade,* p. 171. Harvard University Press, Cambridge, Mass., 1963.
50. Hartnett, R. T. College and university trustees: Their backgrounds, roles and educational attitudes. In *Crisis in American Institutions,* J. Skolnick and E. Currie, pp. 359-372. Little, Brown and Company, Boston, 1973.
51. Servan-Schreiber, J. L. *The Power to Inform: Media—The Business of Information.* McGraw-Hill Book Company, New York, 1974.
52. Marcuse, H. *Repressive Tolerance.* Beacon Press, Boston, 1972.
53. Van Gelder, P., leader of the Baltimore American Federation of Labor-Congress of Industrial Organizations (AFL-CIO). Personal communication.
54. Freidson, E. *Profession of Medicine: A Study of the Sociology of Applied Knowledge,* p. 72. Dodd, Mead, and Company, New York, 1970.
55. Frankenberg, R. Functionalism and after? Theory and developments in social science applied to the health field. *Int. J. Health Serv.* 4(3): 411-427, 1974.
56. Berliner, H. A Larger Perspective on the Flexner Report. Johns Hopkins University, Baltimore. In process.
57. Navarro, V. A critique of the present and proposed strategies for redistributing resources in the health sector and a discussion of alternatives. *Med. Care* 12(9): 721-742, 1974.
58. Green, M. J., Fallows, J. M., and Zwick, D. R. *Who Runs Congress?* Ralph Nader Congress Project. Bantam Books, New York, 1972.
59. Marx, K., and Engels, F. *The Communist Manifesto.* International Publishing Company, New York, 1960.
60. Therborn, G. Power in the kingdom of Sweden. *International Socialist Journal* 2: 59, 1965.
61. *1972 Federal Campaign Finances. Business, Agriculture, Dairy and Health,* Vol. 1. Common Cause, Washington, D. C., 1974.
62. Matthews, D. R. *The Social Background of Political Decision Makers,* pp. 23-24. Doubleday, New York, 1954. (Quoted in R. Miliband, *The State in Capitalist Society: An Analysis of the Western System of Power,* p. 61. Weidenfeld and Nicolson, London, 1969.)
63. Schattschneider, E. E. *The Semi-Sovereign People: A Realistic View of Democracy in America,* p. 31. Holt, Rinehart and Winston, New York, 1960.
64. Titmuss, R. *Income Distribution and Social Change.* Allen and Unwin, Ltd., London, 1963.
65. Kolko, G. *Wealth and Power in America.* Praeger, New York, 1968.
66. Bodenheimer, T. Health care in the United States: Who pays? *Int. J. Health Serv.* 3(3): 427-434, 1973.
67. Rimlinger, G. V. *Welfare Policy and Industrialization in Europe, America and Russia.* John Wiley and Sons, New York, 1971.
68. Sigerist, H. E. *Landmarks in the History of Hygiene.* Oxford University Press, New York, 1956. (Quoted in M. Terris, Crisis and change in America's health system. *Am. J. Public Health* 63(4): 313-318, 1973.)
69. Piven, F. F., and Cloward, R. A. *Regulating the Poor: The Functions of Public Welfare.* Vintage Books, New York, 1971.
70. Committee on Government Operations, United States Senate. *Confidence and Concern: Citizens View American Government: A Survey of Public Attitudes,* Part 1, p. vi. U.S. Government Printing Office, Washington, D. C., 1973.
71. Woodson, D. W. National health insurance: A big role reversal takes place in Congress. *Medical World News* 15(14): 69, 1974.
72. Fein, R. The new national health spending policy. *New Engl J. Med.* 290(3): 137-140, 1974.
73. Glasser, M., Director of the Social Security Department of the United Automobile Workers of America (UAW). Personal communication.
74. Glasser, M. The Pros and Cons of the Private Insurance Involvement in the Health Sector. Paper presented at the Policy and Planning Seminar, School of Hygiene and Public Health, Johns Hopkins University, Baltimore, April 18, 1974.
75. Roemer, M. I., and Mera, J. A. "Patient-dumping" and other voluntary agency contributions to public agency problems. *Med. Care* 11(1): 30-39, 1973.
76. *Washington Report on Medicine and Health* No. 1407, p. 1, June 17, 1974.

PART 3

The Political Sociology of Gender and Functions

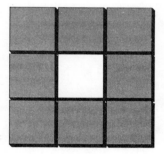

CHAPTER 7

Women and Health Care:
A Comparison of Theories

Elizabeth Fee

What do feminists have to say about the health care system in relation to women? A great deal, and most of what they have to say is highly critical.

Women are recipients of health care, and, increasingly, they have been critical of the form and content of this care. Particularly in those areas of medical care that most directly impinge on women's lives as women—gynecologic examinations, birth control and abortions, sexuality, childbirth, and psychotherapy—feminists have been articulate critics of the nature and quality of medical treatment.

Women are also dispensers of health care. For millennia, mothers traditionally assumed responsibility for the health of their families. Many of these traditional women's tasks have now been socialized, professionalized, and organized in giant medical institutions, but the overwhelming majority of the workers are still female. They occupy the lowest rungs of the medical hierarchy, are poorly paid, and have little power or voice in the organizations in which they work. Clearly, women experience their oppression not only as patients but also within the delivery system itself.

Has a systematic analysis of the relationship of women to health care emerged from the feminist writings of the last decade? Specific complaints are widely shared and generally recognized by feminists, and indeed by women in general, but although they may agree as to the existence and symptoms of a diseased state of health care, the diagnosis of the problem takes several distinct forms. Consequently, different groups may be led to prescribe various cures.

All recognize that women's problems with the organization and delivery of health care cannot be solved within the context of the medical system alone; since this is only one aspect of their social oppression as women, the solutions required must involve more radical social change. One's diagnosis of what is wrong with medical care must be related

115

to one's diagnosis of what is wrong with society in general. Here, not all feminists agree. A feminist consciousness grows from the surfacing of anger at being constantly manipulated, harrassed, limited, and repressed into the social role of "woman"; but the answers to the obvious questions of why this thing happens and how to best struggle against it are not self-evident.

There are at least three forms of social criticism which the women's movement has taken; these may be labeled as liberal feminism, radical feminism, and Marxist-feminism. As these three branches of the feminist movement have differing approaches to the analysis of women's situation, their prescriptions for the ailing American health care system are also different. This discussion of feminism and medicine will therefore be presented in three parts. Each section will briefly describe the general political framework adopted by one branch of the movement and then proceed to a consideration of that group's analysis of medical care. This general and perhaps overly schematic approach is intended for purposes of clarification and also to stimulate discussion; it should be noted that it presents as static positions ones which are in fact highly dynamic and in process of development. Also, although the categories used do describe distinct approaches to the analysis of "the woman question," this is a classification of modes of analysis and not of individuals. Particular women and/or organizations may, and do, adopt elements of each analysis; they may, and do, change their perspective over time, as a result of both external conditions and internal discussion and development. Any attempted description of a dynamic political movement should be out-of-date as soon as it is printed.

LIBERAL FEMINISM

Liberal feminism is the most widely diffused and generally acceptable version of feminism. Even many of those antagonistic to "women's lib" can accept, at least in principle, the goals of equal pay and equal opportunity for women. The liberal feminist position was crystallized by Betty Friedan's now classic text, *The Feminine Mystique,* and given organizational form in the National Organization of Women (NOW); the movement demanded equal opportunity for women to enter the upper reaches of the job market and equal treatment once they got there (1). Liberal feminists do not seriously challenge the hierarchical structure of American society; they simply want access to the same choices as are available to men. NOW fought to "bring women into full participation in the mainstream of American society *now,* exercising all the privileges and responsibilities thereof in truly equal partnership with men" (2).

One of the tasks of this movement was to prove that women were as capable as men, that their exclusion from all the centers of power had no rational or biologic basis. They therefore attacked the nexus of ideas and attitudes, "male chauvinism," that held women to be inferior beings. If women were not *really* inferior, then they were victims of a sexist ideology, supported and reinforced by a system of socialization which trained women to accept and adapt to a limited social role. If the women's problem was not real but ideological, it could be effectively countered by a program that combined persuasion, reeducation, the provision of "role models," and the development of pressure groups which would change both people's ideas of women and the legal and economic discrimination which reflected these ideas.

An underlying assumption was that the chauvinist complex of derogatory feminine stereotypes served no essential social function; chauvinism was either a male psychologic peculiarity or a species of bigotry. It ill served the ideals of equal rights to which democratic societies were supposed to be committed; indeed, it assured the waste of valuable human resources and human talent. It was clearly outmoded, counterproductive, and a vestige of earlier unenlightened eras. The movement would carry on the banners first raised by feminists a hundred years earlier and finally banish the historical hangover of sexual discrimination. The tempo of the sixties favored the belief that equality, or at least the more cautious "equality of opportunity" could be won without the necessity of transforming the economic and social infrastructures of the United States. This considered optimism gained support from a review of their numbers: women were the majority of the population. Unaided if needs be, in alliance with progressive males if they were willing, women could enforce the changes they wanted and needed. In those heady early days few believed that all women did not share the same essential interests or that historical cleavages of class or race might disturb female unanimity. The movement launched a campaign for all the equalities: equal rights in the eyes of the law, equal job opportunity, equal pay, equal access to education, equal promotion and professional advancement, equal credit. Child care and housework—the tangible requirements of the existing order—could be equally shared with men within the family or socially organized in day-care centers and communal living arrangements (3). Future socialization of children into sex-specific roles would be combatted by pressure on the educational system, on publishers of children's books, and on toy manufacturers.

During the flush economic times of the sixties, the liberal feminist movement made considerable headway. The case for equality gained widespread publicity and seemed compelling to many women and men; concrete legislative victories reinforced the belief that gains toward equality were possible "within the system"; they moved on toward a constitutional amendment that would embody their central demand in the fundamental law of the land as their predecessors had done with the women's suffrage amendment fifty years before. The resistance to apparently reasonable demands has proved stronger and more stubborn than the theory would seem to predict, particularly on the part of other women, some of whom cling to women's roles as housewife and mother in preference to the free labor market. Liberals counter with the explanation that women are to have a free choice whether to stay at home or go out to work, but the ideal of free choice seems increasingly implausible in the face of growing unemployment and inflation. Indeed, as the state of the economy has begun to restrict and erode some of the hard won gains of the last decade, many have begun to search for a more penetrating analysis of the roots of their oppression. For many more, however, the direction already marked out seems sufficiently correct and they continue with the struggle to win women's rights and equality within the established system.

Liberal Feminism and the Health Care System

Liberal feminists see the social subordination of women reflected in the sexual structure of the organization of medicine, i.e. in a field where women are the majority of health workers, the upper reaches of the medical hierarchy constitute a virtual male monopoly. The imbalance of the sexes here is more extreme than in most other areas of employment, a situation which seems particularly ironic since the practice of medicine requires personal characteristics compatible with those traditionally ascribed to women. The case of the Soviet Union, where the majority of physicians are female, has been frequently cited to show that no social or biologic necessity enforces the rule that men become doctors and women, nurses. The demand for sexual equality in education and employment should rather result in approximately equal numbers of men and women in each occupational category.

Another area of criticism concerns the nature of the patient-doctor interaction. Physicians heal (or do not heal) from a position of power; they relate in either a paternal or an authoritarian manner to their patients. They may withhold information about a diagnosis, be deliberately vague and obfuscatory, or be simply incapable of explaining the problem in nontechnical terms; they seem to doubt that patients have a right to an explanation of their illness. Aware that these attitudes are also directed at men, liberal feminists correctly argue that they are exaggerated when the patient is female: well or ill, women are accorded less respect. Many women feel that their symptoms are treated less seriously than those of men because doctors harbor the secret suspicion that most of the medical problems presented are psychosomatic.

The "specialist" is a more accurate term than "doctor" to describe the focus of the liberal feminist critique of medical attitudes. Middle-class women usually do not see a general practitioner, but rather a series of specialists: a gynecologist for birth control and pap smears, a pediatrician for the kids' fevers and a psychiatrist for depression and anxiety. The disaffection with medical care, already directed at the upper strata of the profession, tends to concentrate on two specialties: gynecology and psychiatry (4-7). These are the medical areas in which contempt for women is most evident; each has a long history of explicating the disadvantages of a female body and a female mind. A survey of gynecologic or psychiatric textbooks reveals the contribution of medical education to the reproduction of these attitudes in new generations of medical students.

The criticism of the sex-typing of health occupations and that of the sexist attitudes of physicians intersect in the call for more women to be admitted to medical schools. Women physicians should be more capable of treating the health problems presented by women patients with respect, if only because the female body would be less alien and the female mind less mysterious. The overwhelmingly male bias of gynecology and psychiatry would be difficult to maintain if even half of their practitioners were female. Medical research might become less male biased if the research teams were composed of equal numbers of each sex. Rigid distinctions between medical skills and "caring" functions would weaken if they were not reinforced by sexual differentiation; the widespread desire for such an integration is attested to by the popularity of the Marcus Welby image, fictional though it be. Then, too, a feminization of the medical profession and a corresponding invasion of nursing by men would erode the artificial income and status distinctions between doctors and nurses; this relation is maintained as a traditional male-dominant, female-subordinate one.

This liberal critique thus approaches the problems of medical care at the point most visible to the middle- and upper-middle-class consumer, the private office of the physician or specialist. From this vantage point, the giant medical institutions, clinics, and hospital emergency rooms tend to fade from view, although it is here that the health needs of most women are met—or, more frequently, not met. In speaking to the attitudes of male doctors, this critique centers on the tip of the medical iceberg and tends not to deal with the majority of health workers—medical technicians, orderlies, household workers, and practical nurses, over 70 per cent of whom are women (8, 9). In emphasizing the need to equalize the upper ranks of the medical profession by sex, it implicitly acquiesces in a hierarchical structure which rests on a base of exploited, largely female labor. The liberal position offers most to those who can afford a view from the top, to women who might have gone to medical school had admissions been equal to both sexes, to women who would be able to pay for feminist therapy if it were available. It offers less to the woman who cleans the floors of the hospital or is sick because medical care is unavailable or too expensive.

RADICAL FEMINISM

Radical feminist goals are not to achieve equality with men under the existing social and economic structures, but to entirely transform existing social institutions. Liberal feminist solutions seem weakly reformist and inadequate to serve the needs of women; radical feminists do not want to perpetuate a society which is perceived as fundamentally inhuman.

Many of the women oriented toward radical feminism had participated in civil rights, student, and anti-war movements. With radical men they shared certain characteristic ideas and attitudes: a profound alienation from American culture, a distaste for formal hierarchical systems, a contempt for traditional political forms, and a commitment to the radical restructuring of both values and institutions.

It became apparent, however, that existing Left organizations, for all their disaffection from the dominant culture, yet shared one important characteristic with it: sexism. The SDS (Students for a Democratic Society) proved male biased and male dominated; radical women were either invisible or clearly subordinate (10). Most Left women did not object to the idealistic and utopian nature of the New Left but they did want a utopian vision that satisfied *them* as well as their male counterparts.

Even those branches of the Left more firmly based on a Marxist perspective exhibited similar characteristics, some simply grounded in personal sexist attitudes of many radical males, some more deeply rooted in socialist theory and practice. Many Marxists viewed feminism as a bourgeois protest which had nothing to offer a working-class movement except divisiveness. Women's issues, the men would say, should be subordinated to the larger struggle. In any case women would only be able to win their liberation *after* socialism was attained (11). Movement women who looked at .the socialist models held up to support this claim—China, Cuba, and the Soviet Union—found at best a mixed record on women's rights. On a theoretical level, too, Marxist analyses seemed inadequate to explain the particular oppressions of women; Marxist emphasis on the production of commodities in the workplace seemed to slight women's work, e.g. raising children, keeping house. Left intellectuals did not provide a satisfactory theoretical account of love, marriage, the family, reproduction, sexuality, the socialization of children. The canon's basic text, Engels'*The Origin of the Family, Private Property and the State* (12), seemed insufficient (13).

Some of these women abandoned Left organizations, formed independent movements, and developed alternate theoretical perspectives; they attacked those who remained behind as "politicos" who subordinated their own interests as women to male-defined politics (14).

Radical feminists then began producing studies of specific aspects of women's oppression in the United States (2, 14). They analyzed and attacked the patriarchal family. Not only did it directly oppress women, but it socialized children into an artificial and destructive sexual polarization (15). They attacked Freudian psychoanalysis, calling it the ideological basis of patriarchal control, and a justification of the patriarchal family (16). They undermined the conventional model of female sexual passivity, another prop to patriarchalism (17, 18). They dismantled prevailing assumptions about the naturalness and universality of the patriarchal family via historical examinations and anthropologic investigations of matriarchal mythology, rediscovering images of women that contrasted sharply with the vapid feminity of social and media acculturation (19, 20).

These approaches shared an implicit or explicit theoretical assumption—that the central oppressive agent of society was the patriarchal family and the set of psychic and cultural structures it created. Kate Millett (16) wrote that "a referent scarcely exists with which it might be contrasted or by which it might be confuted. While the same might be said of class, patriarchy has a still more tenacious and powerful hold through its successful habit of passing itself off as nature." Class and economic revolutions might succeed and still leave "the socializing processes of temperament and role differentiation intact." Feminists planned to attack the psychic structure itself: "the arena of sexual revolution is within the human consciousness even more pre-eminently than it is within human institutions. So deeply embedded is patriarchy that the character structure it creates in both sexes is perhaps even more a habit of mind and a way of life than a political system" (16).

For radical feminists the central struggle of history was the battle between the sexes, not the class struggle of which the Marxists spoke. This theoretical tendency was given full expression in Shulamith Firestone's *The Dialectic of Sex* (21). Firestone claimed that the biologic division of the sexes was the first and most fundamental class division of history; it provided the basis for the later division into socioeconomic classes. Feminist revolution should thus overthrow not only a specific form of social organization (capitalism) but Nature itself. The revolutionary means of annihilation of sex differences would be the transcendence of normal human reproduction through technology; artificial fertilization and test tube babies would relieve the women of the future of the burdens of natural reproduction, thus ending the biologic underpinning of their oppression. Firestone's brilliant analysis of the structures of women's oppression collapsed at the point where she tried to speculate how the contradictions between the sexes were to be overcome. The difficulty with posing sex as the primary contradiction is that it becomes almost impossible to pose any final solution to the problem; one may suggest the abolition of men but usually without much conviction that such a step would be possible or practicable. Firestone's idea of the abolition of natural human reproduction was an original and even plausible solution to the question, if still not a convincing blueprint for feminist revolution.

The emphasis on sexual oppression as the primary contradiction has served several essential functions. It has directed women's attention to their oppression as women and thus focused attention on precisely those areas where women's experience is different from that of men; it was a necessary precondition for exploring that half of human experience which had generally been ignored or passed off as inessential in the literature produced by men.

Nevertheless, the theoretical difficulties of a perspective based on biologic sex as the basis of women's oppression deserve to be emphasized (22). If women are everywhere oppressed by men on the basis of this biologic difference, then how has this situation developed, how is it maintained, and how is it to be overcome? How is a raised consciousness of patriarchal oppression to be translated into a public political movement dedicated to the transformation of concrete reality? Male supremacy can hardly be predicated on physical strength in a society where strength is not a noticeable characteristic of those in positions of power; the ability to have babies is woman's most obvious biologic trait but not one which can carry the weight of women's oppression. Must women give up having babies to be free? Firestone believed so; she represents one tendency within radical feminism, which views women's biology as the enemy of her human freedom. A different, even opposite position is the glorification of women's reproductive ability as the central and most significant aspect of human life. The *Proceedings of the First International Childbirth Conference* (23) provides a range of views and experience supporting this perspective which has been further popularized in the movement for natural childbirth and breast-feeding as women's most sensual experiences (24, 25).

If the Firestone view seems to slight women's special human contribution in reproduction, the resurrection of childbirth as an essential female experience offers no way out of the impasse. Rather, it seems to return women's attention to the same social roles which can only be experienced as imprisonment within the structures of present social reality.

If the theoretical work of the radical feminists has been uneven, it has been productive in actual struggles against an oppressive reality, and inventive in developing new forms of resistance. In addition to their demystification of paternalist ideology, women have created special organizational structures to combat specific symptoms of their oppression. Among these are the consciousness-raising group, the women's center, the rape crisis center, the women's commune, and the self-help group.

Within these structures women have experimented with different organizational forms, with or without formal authority or recognized leadership; they have sought to break down barriers between women and base their relationships on collective responsibility and mutual support rather than on competition and individual isolation. The thrust has been not so much to demand equality of opportunity in a system known to be structurally oppressive, but rather to organize women collectively, and arm them with ideological tools, so that they may resist their oppression politically. Their general solution is organized, knowledgeable self-defense, backed by a newfound pride in their sex, its history, and its culture. A possible drawback to the small-group strategy may be that it restricts the struggle to the margins of the established order, or leads to the development of alternative enclaves within it. As a political form, the small group may not allow development of sufficient power to confront or overthrow the dominant structures but it aids the development of a collective consciousness and helps to break down the dominant ideology. Thus the ideas of radical feminism have spread from a strong base in the United States and have influenced the development of feminism throughout all Western capitalist countries where the special oppression of women is being explored and rejected. The separate organization of women and the development of both consciousness and theory are a precondition—necessary but not sufficient—for the liberation of women.

Radical Feminists and Health Care

Radical feminists see the medical profession as yet another system which conforms to the patriarchal pattern established in the family. The doctor-father runs a family composed of the nurse (wife and mother) and the patient (the child). The doctor possesses the scientific and technical skills and the nurse performs the caring and comforting duties; these roles, of course, replicate relations within the patriarchal family.

This perspective helps both patients and medical workers make sense of the attitudes they encounter and the feelings they experience when they confront physicians. Visiting a doctor *is* indeed an infantilizing experience; nurses *are* often treated as wives.

What then is the radical feminist solution to health care problems? It is not simply to increase the percentage of female doctors. Radical feminists would agree that it is difficult for a woman to be as authoritarian as a male doctor (if for no other reason than that patients will expect her to be more sympathetic and understanding). But they also realize that women doctors are likely to be socialized into the "physician role" as long as the role itself remains unaltered. Paternalism and authoritarianism are not genitally but structurally and culturally determined. Nor do radicals recommend the construction of health "teams" as an antidote. That solution might simply produce a polygamous rather than a monogamous family; if the patriarchal structure stays intact, then each new health worker would be socialized into the submissive female role. Studies of the roles played by members of existing health teams bear out this suspicion (26). In addition to their criticism of the power of physicians and hospital administrators, radical feminists work to increase the knowledge and thus the ability of patients to resist their infantilization at the hands of those who possess that knowledge. Rather in the manner of the Naderites, they seek to inform and organize those who receive health care and thus indirectly bring pressure on the patriarchs of the system (27).

Radicals argue that women should understand their bodies and know what reasonably to expect from physicians. Only then can they judge for themselves the competence of the care they receive. When dealing with physicians (as when dealing with auto mechanics) knowledge is power. Women are encouraged to press their doctors for information about the results of tests, to draw up lists of questions to ask gynecologists, to acquire their own medical records, to get names of drugs being given, to sit in on medical conferences. Aware that this path is a difficult one—the disparity in specialized knowledge is enormous—feminists call for the formation of medical consciousness-raising groups. The self-help groups of women meet regularly to explore health problems, to share knowledge and experiences about the health system, to become familiar with their own and each other's bodies, to aid one another in following their own cycles by self-examination, to generate an understanding of the normal variations among healthy women in order to facilitate the recognition of symptoms of illness, and to break through the body-alienation imposed on females by patriarchal culture.

The self-help movement started with women's sexual and reproductive functions, the areas of maximum alienation between women and the health system. Members learned to view their own and one another's cervixes, using a simple and inexpensive (50 cents) technologic device, the plastic speculum. This simple self- and mutual examination proved a revelation for many women who had assumed that the impersonality of the routine gynecologic exam—being draped with white sheets, probed by cold metal instruments, surrounded by secrecy and embarrassment—was somehow inherent in the process. The self-help group atmosphere of gentleness, warmth, and mutual support made clear that this too was just another by-product of the existing order. Self-help groups in fact allow the potential patient to make great progress in understanding her own body, and she becomes immeasurably strengthened in future dealings with professional physicians (28).

Another aspect of the radical Women's Health Movement was the development of protest against the American way of childbirth. Normal hospital procedures for expectant mothers are among the most inhumane of medical practices. The prone position, the impersonality, the shaving and probing, the enemas and the drugging, the isolation and the labor inducement, the expense, the enforced passivity—all these lead to misery for the mother and often physical impairment for the infant. Feminists have been articulate critics of this system and have called for the legalization of midwifery, and many have argued that the best way to give birth is at home with husbands and relatives present (23, 29).

As the feminists confronted the intransigence of the health care system, they turned increasingly from consumer resistance to the construction of alternate modes of health care—the women's health centers. These institutions, set up and controlled by women, seek to help women with their health problems *outside* the established institutions. In the women's clinics patients learn about their bodies; they are not turned into passive recipients of treatment. Information is shared and the patient retains control over essential decisions concerning her own health. Education, moreover, is reciprocal: the "providers" seek to learn from the "consumers." Patients may sometimes keep their own records. Care is free whenever possible, or a sliding scale of fees is arranged. Some clinics choose to give free health care by charging for abortions; the income so obtained pays for the running of the entire clinic (30). The Feminist Women's Health Center in Los Angeles is the model for many others. It offers self-help clinics, gynecologic exams and treatment, pregnancy screening and counseling, and paramedical training programs, and it has its own abortion clinic. All staff members participate to some extent in decision making; "directorship" depends on degree of commitment to the health center and the length of time worked (31). In line with the ideal of sharing rather than restricting medical knowledge and skills, there is a summer session to train women to staff other women's health facilities (32).

As radical feminists moved to develop the women's centers as a widespread alternative to the established medical order, they ran into roadblocks imposed by that very system. Increasingly they began to confront the same sorts of problems that confronted the communes, problems inherent in any attempt to organize real alternatives while the old order remains intact, powerful, and in command of the wealth, resources, and political and legal mechanisms of society.

For one thing, there are not enough women doctors to fill the demand. Many clinics have had to rely on male physicians to perform abortions while seeking to retain control and policy-making power in the hands of women. There is a real tension, however, between the power that comes from the possession of knowledge (in this case, medical expertise) and the desire to keep power in non-expert hands. More generally, the radical dictum that knowledge is power itself points to the difficulties inherent in a virtual monopoly of specialized knowledge by the established order. Lack of credentials and shortage of funds make it difficult to obtain access to sophisticated technology and difficult to obtain necessary drugs.

The profession, too, is not loath to defend itself from what it correctly perceives to be a threat to its power and prerogatives. Legal charges of practicing medicine without a license are an available weapon; three women midwives were arrested in March 1974 for their work at the Santa Cruz Home Birth Center on such charges (33). The use of legal restraints to prevent women from carrying on self-help activities has generally failed if only because of the difficulty of deciding the exact point at which an individual's control over her own body is superseded by the restriction of medical practice to licensed professionals. Nevertheless, economic pressures can be brought to bear. The Women's Health Clinic in Portland, Oregon was to have been partially supported by the Office of

Economic Opportunity, but funds were cut because the women refused to set up the proper hierarchy, and had decided to operate the clinic without a doctor (30).

The most important limitation of the radical feminist program for remaking health care is that it deals only with those areas where women's health needs are different from those of men. But a woman's health needs are greater than the care of her reproductive system. The very advances of the women's clinics have only pointed up the obvious shortcomings of the rest of the health care system. Some clinics have attempted to move ahead, and have begun counseling in nutrition and drug problems, but it is manifestly impossible—without a nationwide reordering of health priorities for men and women—for these clinics, operating on the margin of a powerful (though ineffective) health establishment, to cope with all health problems. Women are thus forced back into reliance on the established and unsatisfactory order.

The various feminist alternatives have therefore demonstrated the depth of the difficulties; they have become—in addition to forms of self-help—arenas of political development. Thus Ellen Frankfort complained (in *Vaginal Politics*) that the self-help group was medically dangerous. The flood of congratulatory mail she received from doctors demonstrated to her that they were in fact much more upset at the potential independence the groups afforded women, than over any potential medical dangers. On that score she realized that the doctors themselves had conflicting opinions—profound disagreements—about the medical "facts" in question. This forced her to question her earlier uncritical appreciation of medical expertise (4, pp. 202-204).

The potential of the Women's Health Movement depends not only on the extent to which it is able to provide a more human and less alienating context in which women may learn about their bodies, but also on its role as a model for general health care (34). Thus, its success may increase the awareness among health consumers of the deficiencies in other areas of health care and increase the pressures for a more human and humane reordering of medical priorities. The demand for more consumer knowledge and control over the health delivery system develops as that system becomes increasingly alienated from the needs of the people whom in theory it exists to serve.

MARXIST-FEMINISM

Marxist-feminists have tried to understand the position of women by utilizing the method of analysis developed by Marx and Engels, believing that this is the most effective tool available for understanding all social contradictions, including the oppression of women. They see the essential task of theoretical development within the Women's Movement as that of bringing together feminist consciousness with the historical and dialectical method of analysis.

According to Engels: "We make our history ourselves, but in the first place, under very definite assumptions and conditions. Among these the economic ones are ultimately decisive" (35). Thus, for example, even that most biologic function, reproduction, is ultimately governed by the existing economic structure, as is evident when one looks at the research, distribution, and control of contraception on a national or international level. This is not, however, to say that there is a simple cause and effect relationship between economic structures and human experience and action; in a dialectical relationship, women (and men) both form and are formed by the conditions of their existence. This interaction is a dynamic and evolutionary one. Thus, the development of the mode of production erodes old patterns of social organization which must be gradually, and perhaps painfully, destroyed, and replaced by new patterns adapted to and made possible by the changed economic organization.

Engels (36, p. 618) emphasized that the dialectical mode of thought was not simple determinism:

> Cause and effect are conceptions which hold good only in their application to individual cases; but as soon as we consider the individual cases in their general connection with the universe as a whole, they run into each other, and they become confounded when we contemplate that universal action and reaction in which causes and effects are eternally changing places, so that what is effect here and now will be cause there and then, and vice versa.

Marxist-feminists believe this conception to be of use in exploring and explaining the changes in women's status and consciousness in relation to the development and organization of capitalism.

Sexism has historically been useful to capitalists. Patriarchal assumptions about women's special social role as wife and mother support and reinforce the system whereby women are almost invariably paid lower wages than men for the same work. This system has other functions: it has the effect of depressing wages in general, of increasing profit margins, and of dividing the labor force along sex lines. Yet the very fact that women's labor can be bought more cheaply frequently leads to an employer's preference for female over male labor, especially in the newer areas of mass employment such as clerical and service work. Women are then increasingly drawn into the work force, a fact which in turn undermines the structure of the patriarchal family. Whether the woman has entered the labor force in search of a career and personal fulfillment, or whether she has been unwillingly compelled to do so by the pressures of inflation and male unemployment, the result in either case will be a weakening of the patriarchal family bonds. The wife who is no longer completely economically dependent on her husband can afford to challenge his authority when it runs counter to her own interest. Nancy Seifer (37) has recently provided a sympathetic description of some of the changes in women's consciousness which are occurring in white working-class communities and the increased community activism which is one of the consequences. Other consequences of the increased employment of women outside the home include the increased consumption of prepared foods, the growing demand for day-care centers, and a rising divorce rate as marriages prove unable to adapt to the new social reality.

A division of labor which once appeared natural or inevitable no longer appears reasonable to many women (36, p. 623):

> The growing perception that existing social institutions are unreasonable and unjust, that reason has become unreason and right wrong, is only proof that in the modes of production and exchange changes have silently taken place with which the social order, adapted to earlier economic conditions, is no longer in keeping. From this it also follows that the means of getting rid of the incongruities that have been brought to light must also be present, in a more or less developed condition, within the changed modes of production themselves.

The women who are abandoning their earlier social definitions as protected and dependent wives and mothers are in turn led to demand equal pay and employment as the patriarchal ideology loses its force and social content. Whether the wage differential between men's and women's work will tend to increase or decrease is important for the relationship of feminism to socialism because it will determine the extent to which the labor force will be split along sex lines. Braverman's analysis (38) suggests that while the trend is toward an equalization of labor force participation rates between men and women, the polarization of income will increase as women are concentrated in the lowest paid sectors of employment. The rejection of the sex-typing of occupations by an organized feminist movement and the campaigns against sexual discrimination in employment may, however, impede this development. The support of the Equal Rights Amendment by organized labor is also significant.

What are the historical sources of women's oppression and which structures are responsible for maintaining the ideology of sexism? While Marxists tend to agree in identifying the family as the immediate source of sexual oppression, they see the form of the family as ultimately determined by the nature of economic development and the "social relations of production." Thus Engels in *The Origin of the Family, Private Property and the State* correlates the beginning of women's oppression with the rise of private property and class exploitation. He argues that in primitive cultures males and females divided the tasks, the women gathering and preparing the food, the men hunting; this division of labor was initially reciprocal and not exploitative. With the use of tools, the domestication of animals, and the development of property rights in herds and land (both in the man's domain), the male sphere expanded rapidly in power and importance. Men who now owned the sources of wealth required monogamous marriage to guarantee an orderly inheritance of private property. With the rise of capitalism and class divisions, the oppression of women received further economic underpinning. Almost all males and females came to work for some males, not because the latter group was male, but because it owned the means of production. The working-class family, which still exhibited the sexual division of labor, was always in a precarious financial position. The male laborer was responsible, as Eleanor Leacock (39) writes, "not only for his own maintenance but also that of his wife and children. This to a large measure insured not only his labor, but also his docility; it rendered him—as he is to this day—fearful of fighting against the extremities of exploitation as endangering not only himself but also his wife and his dependent children." To the male fears that stem from responsibilities as breadwinner in a class society are added the fears of increased competition from "liberated" women for scarce jobs. This economic insecurity which Guettel (40, p. 14) terms "the heart of male chauvinism" serves the interests of the owners of capital.

But as capitalist development shifts more and more areas of women's labor outside the family, it undermines the basis of home production. It therefore provides the material conditions for a future abolition of the distinctions between women's and men's work: the cooking of food and the making of clothes are functions which are increasingly absorbed by factory production while the state conducts the unprofitable business of the socialization of children. The development of the technology of contraception holds the potential for women to control their own reproduction (41):

> As long as reproduction remained a natural phenomenon, of course women were effectively doomed to social exploitation. In any sense they were not "masters" of a large part of their lives. They had no choice as to whether or how often they gave birth to children (apart from precarious methods of contraception or repeated dangerous abortions); their existence was essentially subject to biological processes outside their control.

The potential for the eradication of sexual inequality is, however, realized only to the extent that serves the development of capital, and women are the victims of the contradictory requirements which result. Domestic labor within the family serves the production, maintenance, and reproduction of labor power; this essential labor is unpaid yet socially necessary and the arrangement serves the stabilization of capitalism (42-44). Yet women also serve as a convenient reserve labor force. The family burden puts a woman at a disadvantage when she enters the work force (which, if she is a member of the working class, she must frequently do if her family is to survive economically); she is "unprepared, untrained, limited by the children's schedules, etc., [so she] tends to have to settle for what job she can get, and capitalists have always taken advantage of this" (40, p. 54). Women receive lower pay for the same work or are shuttled into low-paid service jobs, particularly those which are motherlike in character (social services, education, health care). Women's wage labor is widely utilized during periods of economic necessity (e.g. wartime) and the women are then pushed back into the family when no longer required. Thus day-care centers may be provided when an influx of women into the labor force is deemed necessary, only to disappear again when economic conditions change. Marxist-feminists conclude that although capitalism has developed a material base for the dissolution of the patriarchal family and the liberation of women, the final steps cannot be taken toward that goal as long as the production and property relations of capitalism remain intact. It is not, therefore, a set of ideas that stands between women and freedom, but an actual concrete set of institutions and relations.

Guettel (40, pp. 25-26) can agree with Millett that male chauvinism is a deeply rooted psychic structure. But from whence do those structures come, she asks?

> For a Marxist, consciousness is not transmitted autonomously from the minds of one generation to those of the next. Psychic realities are always bound to the social and production relations of a society, through social institutions, including the family, that are created out of very real material needs . . . True, masculine-feminine character patterns are far-reaching and will take generations to eliminate, but that is because they are based on a male-female division of labor, the elimination of which requires the transformation of not only the forces and relations of production but also the vast superstructure of social institutions.

To summarize, the relationship of capitalism and sexism has been a contradictory one, On the one hand, capitalism has supported and drawn support from the subordination of women. On the other hand, capitalism has eroded the material base on which the subordination rests.

Feminists have sought to strengthen and hasten along the development of the liberatory side of this dialectic. Marxist-feminists support this effort, believing with Marx that while history affords the possibilities, it is up to people to realize them in practice. But Marxist-feminists argue that although feminism may heighten the contradictions inherent in capitalist society, liberation cannot be attained within the framework of this system. Women's gains will remain contingent, dependent, and limited by the repressive side of the dialectic, by the fact that sexism remains useful for capitalism. Gains won, moreover, will often be hollow ones; equal treatment by a profoundly unequal society is not a satisfactory solution. Finally, any significant gains extorted from the system, and there have been many, are vulnerable to capitalism's repeated convulsions and collapses. During depressions, women and blacks are the first to be fired, day-care centers are swiftly shut down, and programs and policies which are not directly system supportive are cut back or eliminated.

Capitalism, many Marxists argue, cannot free itself from dependence on sexism any more than it can transcend class oppression or the pursuit of private profit at the expense of the satisfaction of real human needs. These drawbacks are built-in components. So a necessary condition of the complete liberation of women, Marxist-feminists would say, is the rejection of capitalism and its replacement by a humane, democratic socialism. The example of China, even after all the difficulties are noted, remains instructive. From a history steeped in the most extreme forms of patriarchalism and the most debilitating poverty, China has taken immense strides forward toward equality and prosperity. Chinese women, in particular, have made extraordinary gains in a mere 25 years (45, 46).

In the United States, a new social order would certainly not automatically eliminate sexism. But with full employment, no inflation, socialized medicine, expanded education, free transportation, cheap food and public services, and the elimination of consumerism and the cult of the home, women would be in a far better position to carry on the struggle. Once the constant nourishment and support that sexism received from the warped priorities and material conditions characteristic of capitalism were removed, once sexism's sustenance was withdrawn, women's liberation would finally be capable of attainment.

Marxist-Feminism and Health Care

Marxist-feminists believe that the specific structures of the American health system which are oppressive to women—as workers and as patients—cannot be understood without an analysis of that system as a whole. That system, in turn, becomes fully comprehensible only when it is recognized as one component of a capitalist economic and social structure. Many of the deficiencies of the modern American health system, like those of the education, transportation, and communications industries, flow from its commitment to the imperative of production for profit, rather than the fulfilment of people's needs.

The health system mirrors the priorities and organization of the larger system which supports it, and which it in turn supports, in a variety of ways: in its intense concentration of financial and political power at the top, in its thoroughgoing stratification of its work force by class, sex, and race, in its division of labor and specialization, in its very definitions of health and illness, and in its lack of accountability to the American population whom it theoretically serves. Let us consider these characteristics in turn.

As in other sectors of the American society, power is concentrated at the top, in a handful of monopolistic institutions. One of them, the American Medical Association, was once the undisputed dominant force in the health field. Times have changed, however. As the standard 19th-century capitalist enterprise—the small competitive firm—gave way to the giant monopoly corporation, so too has the undisputed power of the small fee-for-service solo practitioner been overtaken and largely surpassed by new forms of medical organization. As in other areas of the economy, the increasing reliance on large-scale, expensive technology gave the competitive edge to those who could muster the capital resources to obtain the new equipment. Also complementing the pattern in other sectors, the enlightened wing of the rising corporate class in the early 1900s, the Rockefellers and the Carnegies, strove to nationalize, organize, and centralize the medical system; the Flexner Report (1910) was an important milestone in the process (47).

Power now rests with a coalition that includes, in addition to the American Medical Association, the commercial insurance companies, the research and teaching hospitals, and the voluntary and public community hospitals. These institutions are themselves dominated by members of the corporate class, or of the upper-middle class (middle management and professionals), who occupy commanding positions in almost all major American institutions. At the top are the ten largest commercial health insurers (Aetna, Travellers, Metropolitan Life, Prudential, CNA, Equitable, Mutual of Omaha, Connecticut General, John Hancock, and Provident); among them they control nearly 60 per cent of the multi-billion-dollar industry. Their leadership is tightly interlocked with the corporate and banking sectors, and they exert decisive influence on state policy in matters of health care. In the current debate over how to deal with the financial crisis of the health delivery system, they have (with lavish expenditure of funds) managed to so dominate the discussion that nearly all the proposals for action are simply varieties of publicly supported insurance programs. Most would enhance the profit-making capacity of the commercials and further shift the fiscal burden of the health system to working- and middle-class citizens via regressive tax structures (48, 49).

The great teaching and research institutions are also dominated by representatives of the corporate class. In 1970, for example, Columbia Presbyterian Medical Center had a director of Texaco presiding over a major teaching hospital, the president of United States Steel chairing its finance committee, and the president of American Telephone & Telegraph running its planning and real estate committee (50). These institutions train and socialize the people who staff the upper and middle echelons of the health system. They encourage the development of and reliance upon sophisticated medical technology, an extreme specialization and division of labor, and the flow of funds to esoteric research projects (often involving experimentation on poor, minority, or working-class women) (51).

The voluntary community hospitals are controlled by boards composed of upper-middle-class professionals, rather than representatives of corporate capital; doctors, lawyers, and smaller businessmen predominate. Women, members of minority groups, and representatives of organized or unorganized labor are virtually excluded from access to any of these decision-making bodies (52, 53).

Far below the capitalists and the professionals are the lower-middle and working classes of the health industry. The former comprise the nurses and paraprofessional auxiliary and service personnel, representing 54.2 per cent of the total labor force (48). Both groups are predominantly female; the working class includes an overrepresentation of minority groups. These classes are often played off against one another. Middle-ranking groups are given a degree of control over those below them (though they are excluded from the real decision-making bodies above them). The employment of lower-level workers may be used to undercut the bargaining position of the mid-level groups, as, for example, in the mass employment of licensed practical nurses and nurses aides over the opposition of registered nurses (54).

The non-physician workers are divided into over 375 independent occupations, most of them narrow, specific, and rigidly defined, most representing one aspect of the work once done by a doctor or a nurse, most dead-end, low-wage positions, boring, repetitious, and firmly under someone else's control and direction (55). This process of breaking up labor into little bits, each of which may be parceled out to a single worker, is a general tendency of modern capitalism. The fragmentation, as Braverman (38) shows, is not to increase efficiency, but to maximize management control over labor, and to replace highly paid workers with less skilled and thus less costly ones.

Seventy-five per cent of these health workers are women, doing modern forms of traditional women's work. The old female roles of nurturing, caring, cooking, educating, and cleaning have become, under corporate medicine, such occupations as nurse, housekeeper, dietitian, clerk, or technician. Ninety-eight per cent of nutritionists and dietitians are women (55).

If capitalist medicine fragments the organization of work, it also fragments the delivery of health care. First it provides multi-level services based on a patient's ability to pay. It affords very high quality service to the wealthy; shoddy, assembly-line care for the poor. Specialization makes it difficult, at almost any level, to find comprehensive care.

Medical fragmentation rests on the premise that the body is rather like a machine, and can, like any mechanical system, be broken down into interlocking parts for purposes of repair (56). The patient (the whole) —becomes invisible while parts of her or his anatomy engross the attention of different (and highly paid) specialists. Where the patient has no power over the forms of medical care, his or her experiences of pain or illness become much less relevant to the "case" than the pathologist's report. Where there are class, race, and/or sex differences between the physician and patient, the situation becomes still more acute, personal communication still further hindered.

Capitalist medicine reinforces the capitalist order in still other, subtle ways, in its very definitions of health and sickness. Health is defined in terms of the system rather than the individual. The central concern of medical institutions, Dreitzel (57) finds, is whether or not the patient is well enough to go to work. (This orientation suggests why women's illnesses are taken less seriously than those of men; they are not as crucial to the production process. Their ills rarely interfere with their ability to do housework.)

Capitalist medicine, moreover, prefers to concentrate (in research and treatment) upon the "scientific," "objective," organic basis of illness. Thus it evades the social causes of much ill-health, causes rooted in the structure of the capitalist system itself. Vast quantities are spent seeking the organic basis of cancer, but it proves extraordinarily difficult to wipe out known causes of the disease such as cigarette smoking, asbestos dust in factories, or coal soot in mines. Improving health in those areas would require confronting the powerful interests of tobacco companies, asbestos manufacturers, and coal mine operators.

The process of ignoring the social causes of disease becomes self-legitimating. Disease which cannot be given a specific biomedical correlate is defined out of existence. The physician draws his own distinction between a "real" disease—one whose organic basis can be identified by the available technology—and functional or psychosomatic illness in which the patient's experience cannot be legitimated by a laboratory report. Complaints stemming from such environmental factors as poverty, sexism and racism, the nature of work outside and inside the home, crises in housing and education, problems in personal relationships, and the like, can be "treated" only by tranquillizers or placebos. American women consume large quantities of both. (If the patient has enough money, she, or he, may be able to obtain sympathy from a psychoanalyst, but this option is not generally available.)

In addition to defining many forms of disease as "not real," some forms of health are defined as medical problems. Pregnancy and childbirth are, or should be, considered natural and healthy aspects of human life. American medicine treats them as forms of illness, to be removed from the "patient's" control, a development which the radical Women's Health Movement is struggling to reverse.

In medicine, then, as in the condition of women generally, Marxists find crucial contradictions. On the one hand, the possibility of extending superb health care to the entire population exists; we have the knowledge, the resources, and the need. But the social relations of health care, the way in which it is controlled and organized, act as fetters. The needs of the giant insurance companies, the industrial corporations, and the professional organizations predominate.

Marxists believe that a thoroughgoing reordering of priorities is not possible within the present system. Capitalist medicine's internal dynamics point toward still greater concentration of control, still greater subordination of workers, yet more scientific research and sophisticated technology generating greater reliance on capital-intensive medicine, and ever-increasing specialization and dehumanizing division of labor—a poor prognosis for workers and consumers alike. Marxists believe that the only way to liberate the potential for improved care and better preventive measures is to retire and replace the capitalist order with a democratic socialist one.

A final note: many who are developing a Marxist analysis of health care are male. It is imperative that the specific concerns of women be further integrated into this developing analysis. Contributions to the advancement of Marxist theory must come from women, whether they define themselves as feminists or socialists. Men sensitive to the achievements and concerns of the women's liberation movements can also help oppose the systematic bias toward the male sex evident in much of the existing Left literature, a bias that has operated as a barrier between Marxists and feminists. (A case in point is the book *Sexuality and Class Struggle*, which, despite its title, demonstrates no awareness of understanding of the women's movement, a point made nicely by David Fernbach in his review (58).)

Radical feminists are now increasingly confronting the issues of class and race. *Class and Feminism*, a collection of essays by the Furies, a lesbian-feminist collective, is an excellent discussion of class attitudes and behavior within the feminist movement (59). The theoretical development of both Marxism and radical feminism is aided to the extent to which each can benefit from the insights of the other. In the aim to create a healthy system, indeed a society, which exists to fulfil people's human needs, there is, after all, no contradiction between them.

REFERENCES

1. Friedan, B. *The Feminine Mystique*. Dell, New York, 1963.
2. National Organization of Women's Bill of Rights. Adopted at NOW's First National Conference. In *Sisterhood is Powerful: An Anthology of Writings from the Women's Liberation Movement*, edited by R. Morgan, p. 512. Vintage, New York, 1970.
3. Bernard, J. *Women and the Public Interest*. Aldine, Atherton, Chicago, 1972.
4. Frankfort, E. *Vaginal Politics*. Bantam, New York, 1972.
5. Seaman, B. *The Doctor's Case Against the Pill*. Avon, New York, 1971.
6. Chesler, P. *Women and Madness*. Doubleday, New York, 1972.
7. Miller, J. B., editor. *Psychoanalysis and Women*. Penguin, Baltimore, 1973.
8. Ehrenreich, B., and English, D. *Witches, Midwives and Nurses: A History of Women Healers*, p. 1. Feminist Press, Old Westbury, N. Y., 1973.
9. Rossi, A. S. Barriers to the career choice of engineering, medicine or science among American women. In *Readings on the Psychology of Women*, edited by J. Bardwick, pp. 72-82. Harper & Row, New York, 1972.
10. Dunbar, R. *Female Liberation as the Basis for Social Revolution*. New England Free Press, Boston, undated.
11. Waters, M. A. *Feminism and the Marxist Movement*. Pathfinder Press, New York, 1972.
12. Engels, F. *The Origin of the Family, Private Property and the State*, edited by E. B. Leacock. International Publishers, New York, 1973.
13. Schein, M., and Lopate, C. On Engels and the liberation of women. *Liberation* 16: 409, 1972.
14. Firestone, S. On American feminism. In *Woman in Sexist Society*, edited by V. Gornick and B. K. Moran, pp. 665-686. New American Library, New York, 1972.
15. Figes, E. *Patriarchal Attitudes*. Fawcett Publications, Greenwich, Conn., 1970.
16. Millett, K. *Sexual Politics*. Doubleday, New York, 1970.
17. Masters, W. H., and Johnson, V. E. *Human Sexual Response*. Little, Brown and Company, New York, 1966.
18. Sherfey, M. J. *The Nature and Evolution of Female Sexuality*. Random House, New York, 1972.
19. Davis, E. G. *The First Sex*. Penguin, Baltimore, 1972.
20. Dinar, H. *Mothers and Amazons: The First Feminine History of Culture*. Anchor, Doubleday, New York, 1973.
21. Firestone, S. *The Dialectic of Sex: The Case for Feminist Revolution*. Bantam Books, New York, 1971.

22. Magas, B. Sex politics: Class politics. *New Left Review* 66: 69-96, 1971.
23. Tennov, D., and Hirsch, L., editors. *Proceedings of the First International Childbirth Conference.* New Moon Communications, Stamford, Conn., 1973.
24. Niles, N. Trebly sensuous woman. In *The Female Experience,* by the editors of *Psychology Today,* pp. 22-25. Communications/Research/Machines, Inc., Del Mar, Cal., 1973.
25. Tanzer, D. Natural childbirth: Pain or peak experience? In *The Female Experience,* by the editors of *Psychology Today,* pp. 26-32. Communications/Research/Machines, Inc., Del Mar, Cal., 1973.
26. Fry, R. E., Alech, B., and Rubin, I. Working with the primary care team: The first intervention. In *Making Health Teams Work,* edited by H. Wise, R. Beckhard, I. Rubin, and A. Kyte, pp. 27-67. Ballinger Publishing Company, Cambridge, Mass., 1974.
27. Boston Women's Health Book Collective. *Our Bodies, Ourselves.* Simon and Schuster, New York, 1973.
28. Hirsch, L., and Hirsch, J. *The Witch's Os.* New Moon Publications, Stamford, Conn., 1973.
29. Lang, R. *Birth Book.* Genesis Press, Ben Lomond, Cal., undated.
30. Grimstad, K., and Rennie, S., editors. *The New Woman's Survival Catalog,* pp. 71-73. Coward, McCann and Geoghegan Berkeley Publishing Company, New York, 1973.
31. Downer, C. What makes the Feminist Women's Health Center "feminist"? *The Monthly Extract, An Irregular Periodical* 2: 10-11, Feb/March, 1974.
32. Hornstein, F. An interview on women's health politics. *Quest* 1: 27-36, 1974.
33. Hirsch, L. Police bust. Midwives arrested. *The Monthly Extract, An Irregular Periodical* 3:7, March/April, 1974.
34. Reynard, M. J. *Gynecological Self-Help. An Analysis of Its Impact on the Delivery and Use of Medical Care for Women.* Thesis presented to School of Allied Health Professions, State University of New York, Stonybrook, 1973.
35. Engels, F. Letter to Joseph Bloch, Sept. 21-22, 1890. In *The Marx-Engels Reader,* edited by R. C. Tucker, p. 641. W.W. Norton, New York, 1972.
36. Engels, F. Socialism: Utopian and scientific. In *The Marx-Engels Reader,* edited by R. C. Tucker, pp. 605-639, W.W. Norton, New York, 1972.
37. Seifer, N. *Absent from the Majority: Working Class Women in America.* National Project on Ethnic America, New York, 1973.
38. Braverman, H. *Labor and Monopoly Capital: The Degradation of Work in the Twentieth Century,* pp. 392-397. Monthly Review Press, New York, 1974.
39. Leacock, E. B. Introduction to F. Engels, *The Origin of the Family, Private Property and the State,* p. 42. International Publishers, New York, 1973.
40. Guettel, C. *Marxism and Feminism.* Women's Press, Toronto, 1974.
41. Mitchell, J. *Woman's Estate,* p. 108. Vintage, New York, 1971.
42. Benston, M. The political economy of women's liberation. *Monthly Review* 21: 13-27, 1969.
43. Vogel, L. The earthly family. *Radical America* 7: 9-50, 1973.
44. Gerstein, I. Domestic work and capitalism. *Radical America* 7: 101-128, 1973.
45. Rowbotham, S. *Women, Resistance and Revolution.* Vintage, New York, 1974.
46. Feeley, D. Women and the Russian Revolution. In *Feminism and Socialism,* edited by L. Jenness, pp. 113-118. Pathfinder Press, New York, 1972.
47. Kelman, S. Toward the political economy of medical care. *Inquiry* 8: 30-38, 1971.
48. Navarro, V. Social policy issues: An explanation of the composition, nature and function of the present health sector of the United States. *Bull. N.Y. Acad. Med.* 51: 199-234, 1975.
49. Bodenheimer, T. S. Health care in the United States: Who pays? *Int. J. Health Serv.* 3(3): 427-434, 1973.
50. Ehrenreich, B., and Ehrenreich, J. *The American Health Empire: Power, Profits and Politics,* p. 52. Vintage, New York, 1971.
51. Ehrenreich, B., and English, D. *Complaints and Disorders: The Sexual Politics of Sickness,* pp. 76-78. Feminist Press, Old Westbury, N.Y., 1973.
52. Navarro, V. Women in Health Care. Testimony presented before the Hearings on Women and Health Care of the Governor's Commission on the Status of Women, Pennsylvania, 1974.
53. Robson, J. The NHS Company, Inc.? The social consequence of the professional dominance in the National Health Service. *Int. J. Health Serv.* 3(3): 413-426, 1973.
54. Brown, C. A. The division of laborers: Allied health professions. *Int. J. Health Serv.* 3(3): 435-444, 1973.
55. Reverby, S. Health: Women's work. *Health/Pac Bulletin* 40: 15-16, 1972.
56. Rossdale, M. Health in a sick society. *New Left Review* 34: 82-91, 1965.
57. Dreitzel, H. P., editor. *The Social Organization of Health,* introduction, p. xi. Macmillan Company, New York, 1972.
58. Fernbach, D. Sexual oppression and political practice. *New Left Review* 64: 87-96, 1970.
59. Bunch, C., and Myron, N. *Class and Feminism.* Diana Press, Baltimore, 1974.

PART 4

The Political Sociology of
The State Intervention

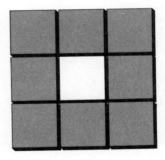

CHAPTER 8

On the Structural Constraints
to State Intervention in Health

Marc Renaud

It is widely assumed that contemporary health problems may increasingly only be solved through the coercive legal powers and fiscal involvement of the state. The state is increasingly called into subsidizing part or the whole of the demand for medical care, into socializing certain costs of the production of care, and into issuing norms and standards for health care delivery, working conditions, environmental controls, drugs, food, and the like. The purpose of this paper is to explore the boundaries of state intervention in health. This essay attempts to identify the structural constraints which preselect the issues to which the state in capitalist societies is capable of responding, and consequently, which set the upper limits on what can be done by the state in order to improve the level of health in the population.

Beyond the most apparent and often nationally specific constraints, such as the existing institutional arrangements, the demands and pressures of interest groups, the electoral platforms of political parties, the national structure of political decision making, and the inextricable problems of management and coordination embedded in a given health system, state interventions in the health field are bound everywhere in the capitalist world by less visible yet real constraints that are deeply rooted in the capitalist mode of production and that are largely above the volition of individual health care workers, public officials, and the citizenry alike. It is argued here that capitalist industrial growth produces health needs that are treated by medicine in capitalist societies in such a way as to make the solutions to these needs compatible with the capitalist organization of the economy. The dominant engineering approach of contemporary scientific medicine equates healing and consumption, that is, in more general terms, health needs and the commodity form of their satisfaction, thus legitimating and facilitating capitalist economic growth despite its negative health consequences.

To the new diseases engendered by capitalist industrial growth, such as ischemic heart diseases, various cancers, and mental and nervous disorders, medicine has evolved an approach which is incapable of acting upon the social component of the etiology of diseases. Illness is reduced to being regarded as a natural process to be treated independently of its social causes by a vast array of experts utilizing the most complex technologies.

When the state intervenes to manage or prevent the crises provoked by some health-related problems, it cannot legitimately overcome the deeply embedded equation between healing and consumption: it can only further commodify health needs. In other words, the cause of the health-improvement ineffectiveness or of the class-biased characteristics of state intervention in the health field must not—although this might be critically important for a given public policy—fundamentally be searched in the Machiavellian wills of some powerful individuals or groups under the control of some medical empire, but must rather be searched in the institutionalized relationships between capitalism, health needs, medicine, and the state, which to an important extent predetermine the potential range of actions of individuals and groups.

HEALTH NEEDS IN ADVANCED CAPITALIST SOCIETIES

In order to identify the boundaries of state intervention in health, the existence of a paradox between "the enthusiasm associated with current developments and the reality of decreasing returns to health for rapidly increasing efforts" (1, p. 1) must first be recognized. Even though human beings in modern societies are born, cured, checked up, and die in hospitals, surrounded by impressive and costly technical apparatus and a complex division of labor, even though it is widely believed that industrial populations owe their higher health standards to the development of scientific medicine, and even though an unparalleled amount of resources is invested in the health sector, there is an impressive amount of evidence (for example, see references 1-9) which shows that current health standards derive less from new "discoveries" and technologies than from the evolution of the environment within which human beings are living, and that current scientific medicine produces more comfort than actual health. In this context, resource allocations to health care seem to derive more from beliefs and traditions, than from evidence of their social utility. A brief overview of the impact of medicine on infectious and chronic diseases will substantiate this assertion.

As Dubos (4) has shown, the great advances in health in the 18th and 19th centuries were largely the result of social reforms that alleviated some of the pollution, dirt, poor housing and crowding, and malnutrition that had come from the industrial revolution (6). And although it is generally taken for granted that the introduction of antibiotics and effective immunization campaigns were the key determining factors in the success of the fight against infectious diseases, Powles (1) and McKeown (9) provide convincing evidence to the contrary. As Powles (1, p. 6) writes:

> Whilst this may have been true in particular cases—for example, immunisation against diphtheria—their contribution to the total decline in mortality over the last two centuries has been a minor one. Most of the reduction had already occurred before they were introduced and there was only a slight downward inflection in an otherwise declining curve following their introduction.

He then cites the research of Porter (10) who

> . . . recently plotted, for England and Wales, deaths in children under 15 years attributed to scarlet fever, diphtheria, whooping cough, and measles in the period 1860-1965.

Nearly 90 per cent of the total decline in the death rate over this period had occurred before the introduction of antibiotics and what Porter refers to as "compulsory" immunisation against diphtheria .... The provision of food, sanitary control and the regulation of births have been the three central factors.

Similarly, McKeown (9, p. 32) argues that

... until the second quarter of the twentieth century the decline of mortality from infections owed little to specific measures of preventing or treating disease in the individual. Mortality began to fall before identification of the causal organisms and, with the exception of smallpox whose contribution to the total reduction was small, long before the introduction of effective immunization or treatment.

To be clear, immunization and antibiotics certainly are effective means to intervene in individuals and they have contributed to the almost total elimination of infectious diseases in advanced industrialized societies. The point is that resources have been invested for infectious diseases under the belief that immunization and antibiotics were the central causes of the diminution of mortality and morbidity from infections, while changes in the larger environment were, in fact, the prime causal factors.

The same point is valid for chronic diseases. Despite the constantly reinforced popular support from which it benefits, and the comparatively much higher amount of resources invested in it, the fight of scientific medicine against chronic diseases also seems only to have produced marginal gains in the improvement of health. For instance, in his *Effectiveness and Efficiency,* Cochrane (3, p. 8) calls for more controlled clinical trials to counter the uncritical beliefs in the virtues of modern medicine, pointing out that

... environmental factors alone were important in improving vital statistics up to the end of the nineteenth century and that until the second quarter of this century therapy had very little effect on morbidity and mortality. One should, therefore, forty years later, be delightfully surprised when any treatment at all is effective, and always assume that a treatment is ineffective unless there is evidence to the contrary.

The available evidence, scarce as it is, tends to show that medicine, to a significant extent, is not effective in its fight against chronic diseases. This does not mean that some individuals do not derive some benefit or cure from medicine but rather that, in the aggregate, medicine is far less effective than is generally taken for granted. Haggerty (6) reviews some systematic measurements of the health-maintenance and health-improvement effectiveness of modern medicine. These include a comparison of a costly versus a less costly treatment of myocardial infarction, comparisons of comprehensive medical care programs in the United States with the available care, albeit often fragmented, episodic, and uncoordinated as it is, the effects of the introduction of modern medical care in a primitive society versus the effects of no such introduction, and so forth. He concludes (6, p. 107):

I need to make perfectly clear that I am well aware that we do have some data on the effectiveness of specific aspects of curative medicine—penicillin for pneumonia, antimicrobial treatment of meningitis, drug therapy for essential hypertension and a few other conditions that have been shown by controlled clinical trials to be positively affected by modern therapy. And I certainly do not wish to belittle the very important effects of our role as relievers of pain and distress .... [But] in sum, we can say that there is not much evidence that illness care (which is what most medical care consists of) reduces mortality and morbidity very much. When well organized, it can reduce utilization of expensive facilities such as hospitals and emergency rooms and can reduce other costs such as laboratory and pharmacy without any measurable difference in health status.

Contrary to what is assumed by contemporary medicine, chronic diseases are to an important extent human beings' responses to environmental stimuli and insults. As Dubos (5, pp. 220-221) says:

> Health and disease are the expressions of the relative degrees of success or failure experienced by man as he tries to respond adaptively to environmental challenges, and also to the inner demands created in him by traditions and aspirations . . . . Many, if not most, chronic disorders are the secondary and delayed consequences of adaptive responses that were useful at first, but are faulty in the long run. When evaluated over man's whole life span, homeostatic mechanisms are therefore less successful than commonly assumed.

Specifically, the so-called "diseases of civilization"—ischemic heart disease, mental and nervous disorders, diabetes, and some forms of cancer—are not simply age-related degenerative processes but are, rather, consequences of changes in behavior associated with economic development and of industrialization-induced changes in the natural environment. Powles (1, p. 12) suggests:

> Industrial populations owe their current health standards to a pattern of ecological relationships which serves to reduce their vulnerability to death from infection and to a lesser extent to the capabilities of clinical [both curative and preventive] medicine. Unfortunately this new way of life, because it is so far removed from that to which man is adapted by evolution, has produced its own disease burden. These diseases of maladaptation are, in many cases, increasing.

In other words, our earlier evolution has "left us genetically unsuited for life in an industrialized society" (11), and the costly and technologically specialized medical repair jobs, despite what appear to the layman as heroic efforts, largely seem incapable of coping with it.

Not only is medicine significantly incapable of dealing with the diseases generated by industrial development—except for some diseases and for symptomatic relief—but there is also evidence to show that medicine itself is producing its own disease burden. As Illich (7) has documented, scientific medicine produces damage that outweighs its potential benefits, on what Illich terms clinical, social, and structural levels. Modern professional health care systems are themselves intrinsically pathogenic because of their therapeutic side-effects, because of the deep dependency they create toward medical care, and because they "transform adaptive ability into consumer discipline" (7, p. 34) so as to paralyze all healthy responses to suffering.

THE MEDICAL AND SOCIETAL RESPONSE

The issues then are the following: Why was the major thrust of the medical response to the new "diseases of civilization" to create more and more costly technologies and facilities, given the absence of convincing evidence of benefit and given that there was evidence that changes in the larger environment played the critical role as the prime determining factor for the improvement of health? Why is it that countries invest between five and ten per cent of their gross national product in the health sector, while the very task of curing and preventing diseases is left unaccomplished, in that the most prevalent diseases—especially ischemic heart disease—are increasing and are killing people at younger ages? Why is it that the state supports medicine so heavily if indeed medicine does produce its own disease burden that outweighs its potential benefits?

The answers to these questions are obviously quite complex and they can only be highly tentative, but because they are so critical to understanding state intervention in health, answers must be provided, however incomplete and debatable they might be.

A familiar argument runs as follows. Human beings have always, throughout known history, culturally endowed certain persons with the authority to define health and illness and with the power to alleviate pain and distress, whether these persons be shamans, priests, or physicians, and whatever their objective effectiveness in curing diseases might be. Despite the proclaimed "rationality" and the idealized search for scientific efficiency in advanced capitalist societies, human beings still cannot escape from being frightened by death and sickness, thus building scientific medicine into a myth and investing the various therapeutic facilities with the appropriate rituals and value-content to celebrate this myth, independently of the costs involved and of their objective health-maintenance effectiveness.

Assuming this point of view to be valid, vital questions would remain unanswered: Why, despite its enormous costs, has modern scientific medicine so overshadowed other ways of dealing with sickness? And why have individuals been so isolated and atomized in their search for health? The key answer to these questions lies in the congruence between the dominant engineering approach within medicine and the larger capitalist environment.

Contemporary medical knowledge is rooted in the paradigm of the "specific etiology" of diseases, that is, diseases are assumed to have a specific cause to be analyzed in the body's cellular and biochemical systems. This paradigm developed out of the germ theory of disease of Pasteur and Koch. This theory contrasted with earlier theories based on the idea of human adaptation and which largely formed the foundation for the sanitary revolution in England in the mid-19th century. While the works of Pasteur and Koch helped to prevent infectious diseases, by a paradoxical evolution of history, their paradigm gave support to the idea of specific therapies, from which arose the essentially curative orientation of current medical technologies toward specific illnesses rather than the sick person as a whole, and the belief that people can be made healthy by means of technological fixes, i.e. the engineering approach. This approach basically assumes, as McKeown (9, p. 29) says, that

> ... a living organism could be regarded as a machine which might be taken apart and reassembled if its structure and function were fully understood. In medicine the same concept led further to the belief that an understanding of disease processes and of the body's response to them would make it possible to intervene therapeutically, mainly by physical (surgical), chemical, or electrical methods.

Because of the dominance of this paradigm, the idea was lost that diseases may be caused by a vast array of interlinked factors tied to the environment or, in other words, that diseases may be individually experienced problems of adaptation. The forgotten idea is what many, including Dreitzel (12) and Rossdale (13), call the "ecological" approach to illness.

Examples of the pervasive dominance of this paradigm, however, abound. For instance, as Powles (1) noted, it is significant that medical establishments were surprised that tobacco smoking actually harmed the lungs and caused cancer, and in some cases virtually opposed this idea. Similarly, it is because of this paradigm that medicine

> ... hesitates to call progressive health-compromising processes—such as arterial degeneration, rising blood pressure and tendency toward diabetes—"diseases" because they are associated with a way of life it feels bound to accept as "normal" (1, p. 14).

It is also significant, to give yet one more instance, that the pathogenic effects of drugs are often underplayed.

This view of health and illness is congruent with the larger capitalist environment because it commodifies health needs and legitimates this commodification. It transforms the potentially explosive social problems that are diseases and death into discrete and isolable commodities that can be incorporated into the capitalist organization of the economy in the same way as any other commodity on the economic market. In an incredible tour de force, it succeeds in providing culturally valued solutions to problems largely created by economic growth, and even makes these solutions to a certain extent profitable for capital accumulation and thus for more economic growth. With scientific medicine, health care has grown into an industry which helps maintain the legitimacy of the social order, and which, in part, creates new sectors of production.

With such a paradigm, "society" is epistemologically eliminated as an important element in the etiology of disease, therefore impeding the growth of a consciousness of the harmfulness of economic growth. The engineering approach transforms the largely social determinants of morbidity and mortality into a value-loaded "rational" system of endogenous causes, thus obscuring the extent to which illness depends on socially determined ways of life and on the damaged natural environment, an enlightened consciousness of which would be potentially threatening to the social order.

In addition, with this paradigm, the treatment of disease does not, as in the past, involve the entire individual. Rather, the individual is isolated in the face of his or her sickness with the help of increasingly professionalized "experts," the physicians. This builds an extremely strong tie between the public and the physicians, whose healing powers, precisely because they are more apparent than real, reinforce the belief in the need for ever more expertise, i.e. in ever more consumption of "expert" services. As Illich (7, p. 84) has well expressed, "The patient is reduced to an object being repaired; he is no longer a subject being helped to heal."

Finally, this paradigm stimulates the consumption by physicians of increasingly complex equipment and the prescription of increasingly differentiated drugs. Members of the public, similarly, are stimulated to consume a myriad of specific products that supposedly will keep them healthy—such as vitamins, anti-depressants, and ultra-violet lamps—in an endless search for health which, in the last analysis, profits those who capitalize on it more than it benefits the health of the public.

In brief, the isolation of the individual from his community, the isolation of the illness from the entire individual, the institutionalized expert solutions to health needs, and the endless consumption process that is unleashed, succeed in transforming health needs into commodities that are often provided profitably by economic interest, but which do not ameliorate the level of health in the population.

It remains an open question whether the "diseases of civilization" are tied to industrialization per se or whether they are linked to the specifically capitalist mode of economic growth. Sufficient, direct, and reliable evidence is not available. On the one hand, since these diseases derive from changes in behavior associated with economic development and from changes in the natural environment induced by industry, it is likely that they will be prevalent under industrialization in both its capitalist and socialist forms. On the other hand, however, since socialism, in theory if not in practice in the existing socialist societies, gives precedence to human needs rather than to capital accumulation, it is also likely that these diseases will be less prevalent with socialism. In any case, the key difference between the approaches to health in contemporary capitalist and socialist societies relates more to how medicine can cope with these diseases than to the sheer prevalence of the diseases. Under capitalism, because the engineering model of medicine institutionalizes a self-defeating dependence on economic growth to solve the problems associated with that growth, it is unlikely that viable solutions can be devised and put into effect to correct the conditions giving rise to these diseases. On the contrary, if we may believe certain reports (see, for example, references 14-16), there are signs that certain socialist societies are in a better position to implement a very different approach to health, illness, and medicine. If only because of the ideology behind them, all self-defined socialist health policies are more prone to be responsive to issues such as the qualities of life at work, of food, and of the natural environment.

THE BOUNDARIES OF STATE INTERVENTION

When the state intervenes in the health sector, it has a quite wide range of potential actions, which vary from country to country according to differing institutional arrangements and class relationships, but, everywhere in the capitalist world, the range of state actions is limited by the fact that environmental health needs usually must be transformed into commodities to insure the survival of the capitalist organization of the economy. The state can only aggregate individual needs and social commodity exchanges into national budgets and plans, but it cannot reorganize the economy so that less illness is produced.

The state in advanced capitalist societies is the legitimate problem-solver, in that it cautiously manages crises and develops long-term-avoidance strategies in an effort to fulfil two inherently contradictory functions: to sustain capital accumulation and to legitimize the social consequences of this accumulation. The state has the distinguishing feature of being the ultimate locus where contradictions have to be resolved and social tensions reduced for the social order to be maintained. Yet, the state is not a neutral mechanism. It is not an arbiter between social classes, but an element in the class system itself. It must simultaneously maintain or improve the conditions for profitable capital accumulation, thus inevitably favoring those individuals who profit from this accumulation, while maintaining or improving the conditions for social harmony, i.e. it has to appear as a universal rather than a class-based state (17-20).

In intervening in the health field, the state, then, must be responsive both to the economic requirements of the health industry and to the organized demands of the public. Schematically, there are two possibilities, the one in which a given public policy satisfies both needs and the one in which the demands and requirements do not coincide.

In the first instance the state can relatively easily intervene. This, for example, is the case with health insurance programs. The considerable debates and political struggles which usually surround their enactment are only the public expression of the negotiating strategies of interest groups; they are the political rituals that create the beliefs and the expectations that help interest groups to maintain or improve their powers and privileges. To focus only on these debates and struggles obscures the extent to which much more sociologically important although less directly visible structural constraints and imperatives are at stake; these constraints and imperatives largely predetermine which issues get defined and who wins and who loses in a given confrontation (21). On the other hand, when the economic requirements of the health industry as a whole and the demands of social movements do *not* coincide, the state is caught in a very precarious equilibrium, endlessly searching for legitimizing solutions to ever more exacerbated contradictions and social tensions. To substantiate these hypotheses, let us examine the internal dynamics of state intervention in health.

With the evolution of the medical engineering model toward increasingly specialized and differentiated products and services, the producers and providers of medical goods have gained considerable control over the health sector, to the extent that physicians have lost their entrepreneurial autonomy. Hospitals and drug and medical equipment manufacturers have increasingly become the heart of health care delivery and, simultaneously, these organizations need ever more consumption of their services and goods in order to survive. They require ever more help from the state to maintain or improve the level of consumption, middle-income consumers having been priced out of the market.

With this evolution, various consumer groups and working-class movements filter out the health needs of the population and articulate demands for a more equal distribution of the culturally acclaimed blessings of modern medicine.

Because of pressures from above and/or from below, the state thus has to become responsive to issues of equity of access at a "reasonable" price to the consumer and at "reasonable" costs for its own fiscal capacity. This is what universal health insurance programs are all about: they maintain or improve the conditions for capital accumulation and they recreate social harmony by slightly redistributing income. Paradoxically, they may be interpreted both as a "victory" for the working class, which "wins" easier access to medical services, and as a "victory" for the medical care producers, because of the benefit they get from increased consumption. That the use-value of such programs for satisfying the health needs of the population be nil is not at stake; what matters for the state is their exchange-value for popular support and their use-value for reproducing capitalism.

State intervention to maintain or extend the market for health goods or services automatically politicizes health care delivery and imposes, in the short run, the necessity for some form of regulation—either through its own bureaucracy or through a delegation of state authority—the most important of which being the "planning" of the allocation of resources. Even though no precise norms of "what ought to be" can be agreed upon, the state has to find means to facilitate the geographical and financial access to physicians and to hospitals, and to limit the expensive competition among physicians, among hospitals, and among drug firms, but always with the objective of both satisfying the demand for care and maintaining the overall costs as low as possible.

But these two objectives are inherently contradictory because the demand for medical and hospital care is almost infinite or, more precisely, no country has ever experienced an end to it. It cannot be taken for granted that there is a limited quantity of diseases which, if appropriately reengineered by physicians, would result in a leveling off of the demand for care. The cause of this situation is not simply that people are hypochondriacs or that physicans only are income-maximizers utilizing hospital facilities as much as they can, but rather that the very medical care that people receive, as well as the very machinery used by physicians in hospitals, help to produce more comfort than actual health. Modern medicine does not deal with the environmental stimuli and insults which are the prime causes of disease; in fact, overmedicalization produces new diseases. In their search for health, people and physicians alike are thus led into constantly more consumption: more physician visits, more pills prescribed, more laboratory tests, and more surgery. And the state has to find means to limit this increasingly expensive and partially health-damaging consumption.

Once the state subsidizes the consumption of medical care, it is thus caught in the internal contradictions of contemporary medical care. The problems of access inevitably lead to the problems of the costs, organization, and administration of health services.

Because an easier access to care brings about a higher demand for care and thus higher overall costs, and/or because of social movements clearly identifying and publicizing some health-damaging environmental conditions, the state may become concerned with issues related to the health-maintenance or health-improvement effectiveness of the health industry. This is where the structural constraints imposed by the economically determined equation between health needs and the commodity form of their satisfaction are more felt. The state is confronted by forces hopelessly outside of its reach.

The state cannot act against the alienation built into the work process in capitalist economies, even though the quality of the work process might be a prime determinant of diseases. As a Special Task Force to the Secretary of the Department of Health, Education, and Welfare recently noted in a report entitled *Work in America* (22):

> In an impressive 15-year study of aging, the strongest predictor of longevity was work satisfaction. The second best predictor was overall "happiness" . . . . Other factors are undoubtedly important—diet, exercise, medical care, and genetic inheritance. But research findings suggest that these factors may account for only about 25% of the risk factors in heart disease, the major cause of death. That is, if cholesterol, blood pressure, smoking, glucose level, serum uric acid, and so forth, were perfectly controlled, only about one-fourth of coronary heart disease could be controlled. Although research on this problem has not led to conclusive answers, it appears that work role, work conditions, and other social factors may contribute heavily to this "unexplained" 75% of risk factors.

In its intervention, the state in capitalist societies cannot act directly or indirectly against the poor quality of work without threatening the accumulation process on which its own survival in part depends. It cannot question the basic factor that makes work unhealthy: the fact that workers largely are only commodities utilized for maximum output, efficiency, and profit. It can only act on very limited, discrete, and easily identifiable working conditions.

The state cannot eliminate the artificial opulence created by capitalism; it can only publicize the needs for dieting and exercising, and for not smoking or drinking alcohol. It cannot stop automobile accidents; it can only coerce car manufacturers into engineering better cars and enforce the obligation to wear safety-belts. It cannot eliminate the unhealthy comfort of our ways of life; it can only better analyze and regulate the production of drugs and food. It cannot eliminate the factors which account for the differential mortality and morbidity among social classes; it can only try to reduce the effects of some of them. It cannot suppress industries because people have too many accidents or because too many people die within them; it can only force workers to be more careful or provide incentives for the elaboration of better protective devices or of better machines. It cannot eliminate the competitiveness which is stereotyped as successful even though it is a prime determinant of heart disease.

In brief, the state cannot reorganize the economy and correlated life-styles so as to really provide solutions to health needs. At the limit, it can only try to compensate directly for the problems generated by capitalist economic growth, rather than indirectly through health services. If the state gets involved in this more direct form of compensation for health needs, it may intervene in three general directions that are compatible with capital accumulation in the economy as a whole, although they may not be congruent with accumulation in specific industries. They are discussed here in order of increasing difficulty of operationalization.

The first and easiest is to put the blame for bad health on the individual. And it can be done in many ways: by enforcing occupational health policies premised on the idea that most work-related health problems are due to workers not being careful enough, not wearing the appropriate protective devices, and so on; by establishing publicity campaigns to encourage the public to diet, to exercise, to relax, to quit smoking and quit drinking alcohol; by legally enforcing the wearing of safety-belts in automobiles; by evolving programs of immunization, screening, and follow-up. All these policies focus on individual at-risk behaviors and all have in common the imputation of responsibility on the individual. As McKinlay (23, p. 18) well describes it:

> [Individuals] are *either* doing something that they ought not to be doing, *or* they are not doing something that they ought to be doing. If only they would recognize their individual culpability and alter their behavior in some appropriate fashion, they would improve their health status or the likelihood of developing certain pathologies .... To use the upstream-downstream analogy, one could argue that people are blamed (and, in a sense, even punished) for not being able to swim after they, perhaps against their own volition, have been pushed into the river by the manufacturers of illness.

State actions on at-risk behaviors are highly congruent with the bourgeois liberal vision of society according to which well-being derives from individual achievement, poverty from individual failure. They also do not challenge capital accumulation in other sectors of the economy, nor do they threaten the legitimacy of current medicine. On the contrary, such policies favor the development of whole new industries (e.g. diet foods, exercise equipment, differentiation of cigarette filters), and they, if successful, permit a more profitable utilization of a more healthy labor force. Moreover, the policies provide a highly valuable and strong argument to physicians when they cannot deal with, or explain, a given case. Rather than admit the weakness of the engineering model with which they work, they easily can blame the individual for his or her health problems.

A second avenue that the state can take concerns what McKinlay calls the "manufacturers of illness." This is a much more difficult, and thus a less frequent, type of intervention because it allegedly may, in the short run, threaten capital accumulation in some actually profitable sector of the economy. Moreover, because of the interests involved, it cannot come about without considerable input from working-class movements. The state can provide various incentives, e.g. socialization of certain costs, charges for consumption, and establishment of long-term norms, in order to stimulate the development of anti-pollution devices, of better designed machines, of better occupational protective devices, of alternative chemical processes, and so on. Or, it can attempt to regulate certain industries, in particular food and drugs. But, in all cases, the state is self-defeatingly dependent upon economic growth to solve the problems associated with such growth. It is assumed here that new changes in technologies alone will improve the environment; yet, these new technologies might themselves bring new health problems that will again require new technological improvements, thus creating new problems.

A third possible avenue for the improvement of health through state actions is ultimately only possible in socialist societies, although some minor changes can realistically be expected within capitalist economies. It involves the implementation of an altogether different approach to health, disease, and medicine: in brief, the de-commodification of health needs leading to a more direct and intense preoccupation with the social conditions giving rise to disease. Specifically, it involves the development of a new medical knowledge based on what has been called an "ecological" approach, the elimination of the monopoly of the medical profession over the definition and cure of illnesses, the elimination of private property in skills, training and credentials, and a reversal in the actual trends in the allocation of resources toward therapy and prevention, so that human beings can self-produce care of their bodies and minds, individually and socially.

Because the engineering approach within medicine simultaneously legitimates and reinforces capitalist economic growth and, needless to say, its wider organizational and cultural bases, it is intrinsically opposed to such policies. It is conceivable, however, that under certain social conditions, timid efforts could be made to partially implement a new, more preventive and more community-oriented medicine, away from costly technologically specialized hospital-based medical practice. It is conceivable, for instance, that ambulatory care physicians, with more valued ancillary personnel, could become more aware of the need to teach their knowledge, of the global working and environmental characteristics of the milieu where they practice, and of the entire personality of their patients, rather than only focus on their specific diseases in isolation from their community. The barriers that have to be overcome for the attainment of such a goal are very numerous, but not insuperable. The training of ambulatory care physicians has to be refocused, the resistances of already organized interest groups overcome, certain organizational incentives worked out, and so forth.

But state intervention within capitalist economies can only remain limited to the reorganization of a proportionally very small segment of the health sector, and even the health-maintenance or health-improvement effectiveness of such reforms can only be very limited. For, larger forces—which are above the wills of physicians, public officials, and the public *alike*—impose the view that progress, in medicine and otherwise, is the sum total of ever more scientific expertise and technological advances, consumed by more and more individuals in ever greater quantity. Without a reversal in this view of progress and in its infrastructural determinants, it is unlikely that medicine and the social organization of health care will fundamentally be changed.

CONCLUSION

This paper has attempted to explore the general structural constraints which are imposed upon all states in capitalist societies in their problem-solving endeavors relative to health. The general argument has been that capitalist industrial growth both creates health needs and institutionalizes solutions to these needs that are compatible with capital accumulation. The key mechanism in this institutionalization is the medical engineering model which transforms health needs into commodities for a specific economic market. When the state intervenes, it is bound to act so as to further commodify health needs, thus favoring the unparalleled expansion of a sector of the civilian economy to the profit of those who capitalize on it, and thus further alienating individuals from control over their bodies and mind but without a significant improvement in the available indicators of the health status of the population.

It remains to be seen if the current efforts toward improving the quality of life in the natural environment, in working conditions, and in food, and toward implementing a new comprehensive social medicine, can succeed in ameliorating health. The deeply embedded and camouflaged logic of the capitalist social order in health predicts that partial successes can be obtained only at the price of considerable struggle. The conditions of success are embedded in the historically and nationally specific evolution of class relationships and they largely can only be understood in relation to specific political and economic conjunctures (e.g. see reference 24).

Acknowledgments—Earlier drafts of this essay have benefited from the comments and criticisms of Robert R. Alford, Roger Friedland, Sander Kelman, James O'Connor, Louise Roy, and Julia Wrigley. Needless to say, the present version is entirely the author's own responsibility.

REFERENCES

1. Powles, J. On the limitations of modern medicine. *Science, Medicine and Man* 1(1): 1-30, 1973.
2. Boyden, S. V. Cultural adaptation to biological maladjustment. In *The Impact of Civilization on the Biology of Man,* edited by S. V. Boyden. (Proceedings of the Symposium of the Australian Academy of Sciences, Canberra, 1968.) University of Toronto Press, Toronto, 1971.
3. Cochrane, A. L. *Effectiveness and Efficiency: Random Reflections on Health Services.* Nuffield Provincial Hospitals Trust, London, 1972.
4. Dubos, R. *Mirage of Health: Utopias, Progress and Biological Change.* Doubleday, New York, 1959.
5. Dubos, R. The biology of civilization—With emphasis on perinatal influences. In *The Impact of Civilization on the Biology of Man,* edited by S. V. Boyden, pp. 219-230. (Proceedings of the Symposium of the Australian Academy of Sciences, Canberra, 1968.) University of Toronto Press, Toronto, 1971.
6. Haggerty, R. J. The boundaries of health care. *The Pharos of Alpha Omega Alpha* 35(3): 106-111, 1972.
7. Illich, I. *Medical Nemesis: The Expropriation of Health.* Center for Intercultural Documentation, Cuernavaca, Mexico, 1974.
8. McKeown, T., and Lowe, C. R. *An Introduction to Social Medicine.* Blackwell Scientific Publications, Oxford, 1966.
9. McKeown, T. A historical appraisal of the medical task. In *Medical History and Medical Care: A Symposium of Perspectives,* edited by T. McKeown and G. McLachlan, pp. 29-55. Oxford University Press, New York, 1971.
10. Porter, R. R. The contribution of the biological and medical sciences to human welfare. In *Presidential Addresses of the British Association for the Advancement of Science, Swansea Meeting, 1971,* p. 95. (Quoted in J. Powles, On the limitations of modern medicine. *Science, Medicine and Man* 1(1): 1-30, 1973.)
11. Rose, G. Epidemiology of ischaemic heart disease. *Br. J. Hosp. Med.* 7(3): 285-288, 1972. (Quoted in J. Powles, On the limitations of modern medicine. *Science, Medicine and Man* 1(1): 1-30, 1973.)
12. Dreitzel, H. P., editor. *The Social Organization of Health.* Macmillan Company, New York, 1971.
13. Rossdale, M. Health in a sick society. *New Left Review* 34: 82-90, 1965.
14. Horn, J. S. *Away with All Pests: An English Surgeon in People's China.* Monthly Review Press, New York, 1969.
15. Peyrefitte, A. *Quand la Chine s'éveillera . . . .* Librairie Arthème Fayard, Paris, 1973.
16. Macciocchi, M.-A. *De la Chine.* Editions du Seuil, Paris, 1974.
17. Offe, C. Political authority and class structure: An analysis of late capitalist societies. *International Journal of Sociology* 2(1): 73-108, 1972.
18. Offe, C. Advanced capitalism and the welfare state. *Politics and Society* 2(4): 479-488, 1972.
19. O'Connor, J. *The Fiscal Crisis of the State.* St. Martin's Press, New York, 1973.
20. Wolfe, A. New directions in the Marxist theory of politics. *Politics and Society* 4(2): 131-159, 1974.
21. Alford, R. R. Towards a Critical Sociology of Political Power: Political Sociology Versus Political Economy in the Theory of the State. Paper delivered at the meeting of the American Sociological Association, New York, August 1973.
22. Special Task Force to the Secretary of Health, Education, and Welfare. *Work in America,* pp. 77-79. MIT Press, Cambridge, Mass., 1973.
23. McKinlay, J. B. A Case for Refocussing Upstream: The Political Economy of Illness. Unpublished paper, Boston University, 1974.
24. Renaud, M. The Political Economy of the Quebec State Interventions in Health: Reform or Revolution? Ph.D. thesis, University of Wisconsin, Madison, forthcoming.

CONTRIBUTORS TO THE VOLUME

THOMAS BODENHEIMER is a staff researcher at the San Francisco office of the Health Policy Advisory Center. He also works as an internist at South of Market Health Center in San Francisco. A graduate of Harvard Medical School, Dr. Bodenheimer received an M.P.H. from the University of California at Berkeley. He has written extensively on topics related to the politics of health care.

STEVEN CUMMINGS is a medical student at the University of California at San Francisco. He is a former graduate research psychologist in health services research in the Division of Community Medicine, University of California at San Francisco.

ELIZABETH FEE is an instructor in the humanities and archivist at the School of Health Services, Johns Hopkins University. She previously taught in the History Department at the State University of New York at Binghamton. Ms. Fee is currently completing her Ph.D. degree in the history and philosophy of science at Princeton University. She has published several articles on scientific theories about women, and is interested in the history of sexuality and of the family.

RONALD FRANKENBERG has been professor of sociology at the University of Keele since 1969. He was previously lecturer, senior lecturer, and reader in sociology at the University of Manchester, where he received his doctorate in social anthropology in 1954. He came to Keele from the University of Zambia, where he was involved both in establishing a medical school and in research on health and medical care with Joyce Leeson. Dr. Frankenberg's publications include *Village on the Border* (1957) and *Communities in Britain* (1966), in addition to various papers on medical care in Africa and China.

ELIZABETH HARDING is an associate professor in the School of Nursing, University of California at San Francisco. She received a B.S. in nursing from the University of Connecticut and an M.S. at the University of California at San Francisco. She has worked as a registered nurse at Montefiore Hospital in New York, University of California Hospital, and San Francisco General Hospital.

SANDER KELMAN teaches in the Department of Preventive Medicine and Community Health at the University of Illinois Medical Center. He was formerly an assistant professor of medical economics in the Sloan Program of Health and Hospital Administration at Cornell University. Since receiving a Ph.D. in economics from the University of Michigan in 1970, his principal research interests have been in the area of the political economy of health and medical care. He is the author of "Toward the Political Economy of Medical Care," published in *Inquiry* in 1971.

147

VICENTE NAVARRO presently teaches at the Johns Hopkins University. Prior to that, he taught health and social policy, political economy, and political sociology at a number of academic institutions in Spain, Italy, France, Sweden, Great Britain, the U.S., Canada, Cuba, Mexico, Argentina, and Colombia. He is an advisor to several governments and international agencies. A founder of the International Study Group on Political Economy of Medical Care, Dr. Navarro is the author of *Medicine Under Capitalism*. He is also editor-in-chief of the *International Journal of Health Services*.

MARC RENAUD is an assistant professor in the Department of Sociology at the University of Montreal. He received his Ph.D. at the University of Wisconsin at Madison. His doctoral thesis was entitled "The Political Economy of the Quebec State Interventions in Health: Reform or Revolution?"